RHEUMATOID ARTHRITIS DIET COOKBOOK

Learn about the key foods that can help alleviate symptoms of rheumatoid arthritis and support joint health with 28-days delicious meal plan

JESSICA C. STEPHEN

Disclaimer

The information in this book is meant solely for educational reasons. This book's contents are not meant to be used in place of expert medical advice, diagnosis, or treatment. Any decisions you make about your health must be discussed with a licensed healthcare provider.

Every effort has been made by the author to guarantee that the material in this book is correct and current as of the date of publication. Still, since medical knowledge advances rapidly, new studies might be conducted that change our understanding this illness and how best to manage it with food.

This book may contains references to and mentions of various people, things, websites, organizations, and other entities that the author does not support, advocate, or have any association with. There is no implied sponsorship or collaboration; all references and remarks are made only for informational purposes.

In order to address their individual health concerns, readers are advised to independently verify any information contained in this book and to consult with healthcare specialists. Any negative effects arising from the use or implementation of the material in this book, whether direct or indirect, are not the responsibility of the author or the publisher.

The dietary suggestions and counsel provided in this book are broad in scope and might not be appropriate for every individual. Readers are recommended to seek tailored counsel from trained healthcare specialists as individual health problems and demands differ.

The reader accepts the conditions of this disclaimer by reading this book.

FACTS ABOUT THIS BOOK

The "Rheumatoid Arthritis Diet" book is an extensive and priceless tool for anyone struggling to manage their rheumatoid arthritis (RA). It starts by giving a comprehensive explanation of the illness and highlighting how much of an impact it has on life quality. This book lays the foundation for a comprehensive approach to well-being by exploring the complexities of RA and emphasizing the critical role that diet plays in managing the condition.

This book's second part delves into the fundamentals of a diet for rheumatoid arthritis, explaining the complex relationship between food choices and inflammation. It explores the significance of essential nutrients for joint health and pinpoints typical triggers for RA symptoms, providing readers with a basic knowledge of how nutrition may affect their illness.

Building a foundation of vital nutrients—such as antioxidants and omega-3 fatty acids, which have been shown to have anti-inflammatory properties—is a crucial component of this book. It emphasizes the value of vitamins and minerals in the treatment of rheumatoid arthritis, equipping readers with the information they need to make wise dietary decisions.

Beyond theory, this book offers helpful advice on what foods to include in a diet for RA patients. Certain categories are suggested, such as foods high in fish and omega-3 fatty acids, vibrant fruits and vegetables, nutritious grains, lean meats, or plant-based substitutes. This book examines dietary components such as dairy and gluten, as well as their substitutes and sensitivities, acknowledging their possible influence on symptoms and inflammation.

An important issue that clarifies the complex relationship between weight and rheumatoid arthritis is weight control. This book provides advice on how to manage weight healthily, emphasizing the benefits of exercise for joint health.

A variety of useful dietary advice is provided, including meal planning, the best ways to cook food to retain nutrients, and how to make wise decisions when dining out. The importance of supplements in the treatment of RA is discussed, with a focus on the necessity of consulting with medical experts to guarantee a well-rounded strategy.The importance of lifestyle elements on overall well-being is acknowledged and consideration is given to them, such as stress management, getting enough sleep, and engaging in balanced physical exercise.

This book places a strong emphasis on customized diet programs, advising readers to recognize their triggers, keep food diaries as a tool for self-discovery, and see a professional for advice.

There is a thorough discussion of overcoming obstacles and maintaining motivation to follow the diet, taking into account the typical problems people may encounter. This book advocates for the value of establishing connections with supporting communities and encourages a positive, goal-oriented approach to long-term health.

This book goes beyond diet in its last section to offer a thorough management strategy for rheumatoid arthritis. It discusses medicine and treatment choices, the value of working with medical professionals, and all-encompassing methods to improve general well-being. All things considered, "Rheumatoid Arthritis Diet" is an invaluable resource that equips readers with the knowledge and useful techniques they need to effectively manage their illness and enhance their quality of life

Table of Contents

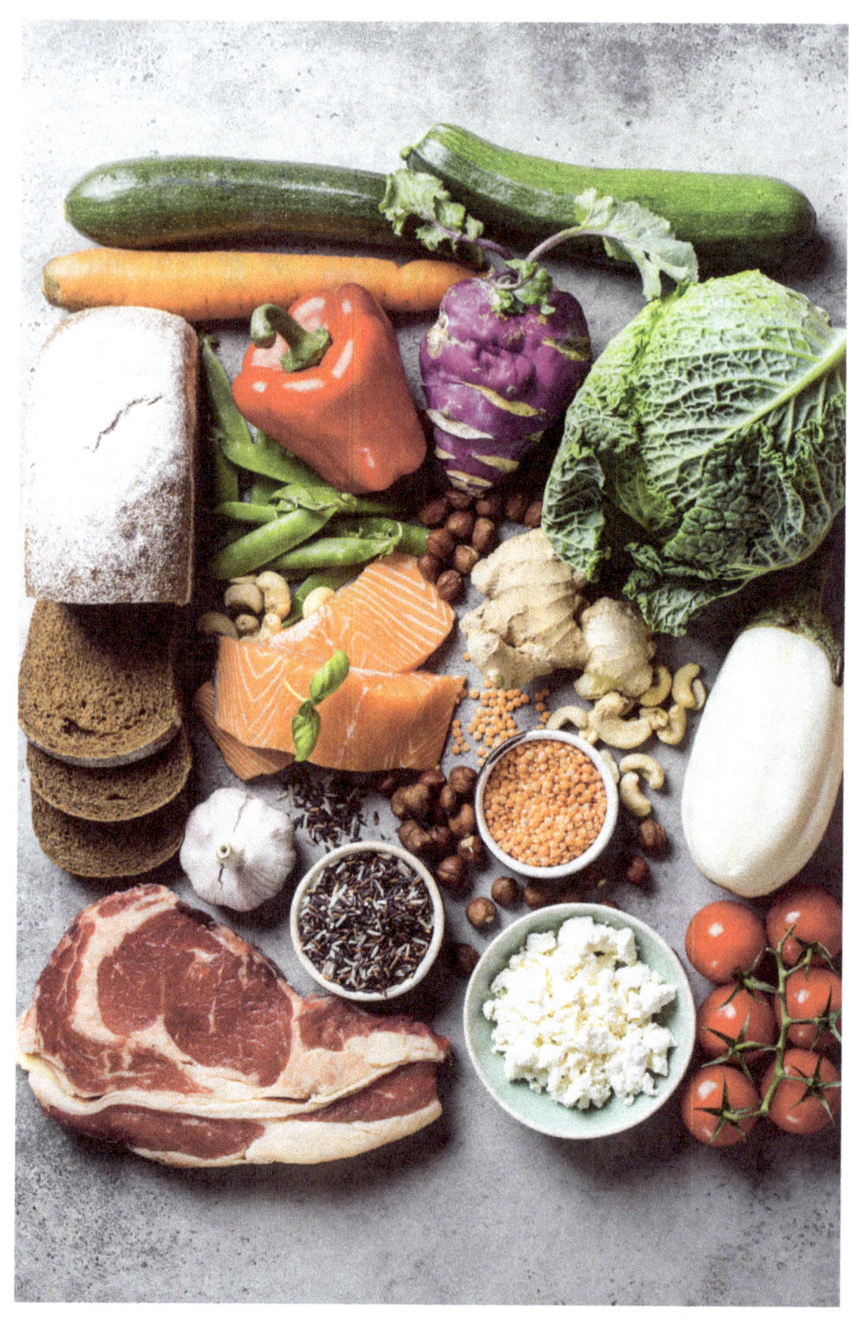

CHAPTER ONE

OVERVIEW OF RHEUMATOID ARTHRITIS

The Basics of Rheumatoid Arthritis

A chronic autoimmune illness mostly affecting the joints, rheumatoid arthritis (RA) causes discomfort, inflammation, and finally joint abnormalities and destruction. The lining of the membranes surrounding the joints, known as the synovium, is attacked by the immune system in the event of RA, as opposed to osteoarthritis, which is the consequence of joint wear and tear. This immunological reaction usually affects both sides of the body and results in swelling, discomfort, and stiffness in the afflicted joints. In addition to harming the joints, RA can also damage the heart, lungs, and eyes.

Although the precise etiology of RA is unknown, it is thought to occur as a result of a confluence of environmental and genetic variables. It frequently shows up symmetrically, affecting matching joints on both sides of the body at the same time. Fatigue, stiffness in the morning, edema, and joint pain are typical symptoms. Being a progressive illness, RA can greatly impair a person's ability to go about their daily life and lower their quality of life in general if it is not properly managed.

Effect on Life Quality

The effects of rheumatoid arthritis on a person's quality of life go far beyond the physical restrictions brought on by stiffness and pain in the joints. Due to the disease's chronic nature and the unpredictable nature of flare-ups, mental discomfort, worry, and despair may result. People who are always battling pain and exhaustion may become socially isolated because they find it difficult to engage in things they used to enjoy.

The effect on productivity and job can further worsen the disease's emotional toll and put a financial strain on the family.

A multidisciplinary strategy for managing RA is frequently necessary, comprising rheumatologists, physical therapists, and perhaps surgical procedures. Since RA damages joints irreversibly, early detection and treatment are essential to reducing long-term effects. Even with new treatment choices, RA is still a chronic illness, and those who have it must manage their symptoms for the rest of their lives and adjust to the disease's ever-changing course.

Dietary Management of Rheumatoid Arthritis

There is no one-size-fits-all approach to controlling rheumatoid arthritis, but diet plays a big part in the process. Although there isn't a single "RA diet," there are dietary approaches that can help manage symptoms and improve general health.

Flaxseeds and fish oil, which are rich sources of omega-3 fatty acids, offer anti-inflammatory qualities that may help lessen stiffness and soreness in the joints. Foods high in antioxidants, such as fruits and vegetables, can also help the body control inflammation.

Furthermore, a few RA sufferers have mentioned the advantages of following an anti-inflammatory diet that lowers the intake of processed foods, sweets, and saturated fats. Rather, emphasis is placed on entire foods with inherent anti-inflammatory qualities.

Furthermore, keeping a healthy weight with a balanced diet can relieve joint pressure, which may lessen discomfort and increase mobility.

To customize food suggestions to their unique requirements and tastes, people with RA must collaborate closely with healthcare providers, particularly dietitians. Although there is no cure for rheumatoid arthritis, nutrition can help manage the condition better overall and work in conjunction with medical therapies to improve the quality of life for those who suffer from it.

CHAPTER TWO

INTRODUCTION TO RHEUMATOID ARTHRITISNUTRITION

The Relationship Between Inflammation and Diet

The hallmark of rheumatoid arthritis (RA), a chronic inflammatory disease, is joint inflammation. The disease's course is significantly influenced by the inflammatory process, which also causes joint degeneration, stiffness, and discomfort. New studies point to a direct link between food and inflammation, emphasizing how dietary decisions may affect the management of RA symptoms.

It is well-recognized that several meals can increase or decrease inflammation in the body. Foods heavy in processed carbs, saturated fats, and refined sweets can exacerbate RA symptoms by promoting inflammation.

Conversely, RA sufferers may find relief and reduce inflammation with an anti-inflammatory diet high in fruits, vegetables, whole grains, and omega-3 fatty acids.

The generation of inflammatory cytokines is a crucial component of the inflammatory response. These signaling molecules are essential for the immune system's reaction, but diseases like RA can cause them to become dysregulated. It has been demonstrated that antioxidants, which are abundant in vibrant fruits and vegetables, might mitigate the impact of these inflammatory cytokines. Including a range of foods high in antioxidants, such as nuts, leafy greens, and berries, in the diet may help reduce inflammation in people with RA.

Furthermore, dietary regimens like the Mediterranean diet have drawn notice due to their possible anti-inflammatory properties. With a focus on whole grains, seafood, fruits, vegetables, and healthy fats, this diet provides a comprehensive strategy for lowering inflammation. A Mediterranean-style diet has been linked in studies to improvements in RA symptoms, such as less pain and stiffness in the joints.

In summary, people who are managing rheumatoid arthritis must comprehend the connection between inflammation and nutrition. Changing to an anti-inflammatory diet high in whole foods and antioxidants may enhance medicinal interventions and improve the way diseases are managed.

Essential Elements for Healthy Joints

For those who have rheumatoid arthritis (RA), maintaining joint health is crucial because the disease predominantly affects the joints, causing inflammation and possible damage. A balanced diet is necessary for good health overall, but certain nutrients are particularly important for maintaining joint health and controlling the symptoms of RA.

Flaxseeds, salmon, mackerel, and other fatty fish are good sources of omega-3 fatty acids, which have anti-inflammatory qualities that may help people with RA. These fats may lessen stiffness and pain in the joints by lowering the synthesis of inflammatory cytokines. Supplements or foods high in omega-3s can be a useful addition to a diet that is RA-friendly.

Another essential mineral for joint health is vitamin D. It affects calcium absorption and bone health, which is important for people with RA because their chronic inflammation may put them at risk for osteoporosis. Maintaining sufficient vitamin D levels can be aided by exposure to sunlight and dietary sources such as supplements or meals enriched with vitamin D.

Not only is calcium necessary for healthy bones, but it also keeps muscles functioning. Because RA patients may become inactive or experience muscle weakness as a result of the disease, it's critical to make sure they consume enough calcium through dairy products, leafy greens, or fortified plant-based substitutes.

Antioxidants like vitamins C and E also aid in the upkeep and repair of tissues, including joint tissues. Nuts, seeds, berries, and citrus fruits are good providers of these antioxidants. Consuming foods high in collagen, such as bone broth, or taking supplements can help support collagen, a protein that gives joints shape.

In conclusion, a diet high in nutrients, such as antioxidants, calcium, vitamin D, and omega-3 fatty acids, can improve joint health and assist people with rheumatoid arthritis in managing their symptoms. Creating a customized diet plan based on each person's needs might be facilitated by speaking with a certified dietitian or other healthcare practitioner.

Symptoms of Rheumatoid Arthritis: Common Triggers

An intricate autoimmune disease that is impacted by both environmental and hereditary variables is rheumatoid arthritis (RA). Although no one meal causes RA, there are specific foods and lifestyle choices that can act as triggers, making symptoms worse and accelerating the disease's progression. For those looking to effectively manage their RA, recognizing and avoiding these common triggers is key.

Consuming meals that cause inflammation is one of the main triggers. Processed meals, which are heavy in refined carbohydrates and trans fats, can exacerbate RA symptoms by inflaming the body. An RA-friendly diet should minimize or eliminate fried foods, sugary snacks, and processed meats to help reduce inflammation.

Another possible trigger is drinking too much alcohol. Alcohol can worsen liver damage and reduce the effectiveness of RA drugs, which is concerning for people who are already managing possible drug side effects. Drinking alcohol is usually advised to be avoided or consumed in moderation by people with RA.

Some RA sufferers claim that the molecules called alkaloids found in nightshade foods like tomatoes, peppers, and eggplants exacerbate their symptoms. Even though the research on nightshades' effects is conflicting, some people may feel better if they cut back on or avoid these veggies altogether.

Wheat and other grains include a protein called gluten, which has been linked to inflammation in certain people, including RA patients. There may be a connection between autoimmune disorders and gluten sensitivity, according to certain research. Those who are having problems with their joints or digestive system can think about investigating a gluten-free diet under a doctor's supervision.

In conclusion, identifying and avoiding typical triggers for rheumatoid arthritis symptoms can be extremely important for controlling the condition. Personalized strategies for managing RA include investigating any sensitivity to gluten or nightshades, reducing alcohol use, and implementing an anti-inflammatory diet in collaboration with their medical team.

CHAPTER THREE

FOUNDATION BUILDING: VITAL NUTRIENTS

Omega-3 Fatty Acids and Their Potential to Reduce Inflammation

Since omega-3 fatty acids have strong anti-inflammatory properties, they are essential for the nutritional therapy of rheumatoid arthritis (RA). Extensive research has been conducted on the potential of these essential fatty acids, which are mostly present in fatty fish like salmon, mackerel, and tuna, as well as flaxseeds and walnuts, to reduce inflammation in the body. Inflammation has a major role in joint pain and damage associated with RA.

Two important forms of omega-3 fatty acids, eicosapentaenoic acid (EPA) and docosahexaenoic acid (DHA), have been demonstrated to inhibit the synthesis of inflammatory molecules, including prostaglandins and cytokines. This inhibition helps reduce swelling and stiffness in the joints, which are symptoms of RA. Furthermore, in certain people, omega-3 fatty acids may lessen the need for anti-inflammatory drugs by improving joint function.

Furthermore, these fatty acids have the potential to slow down the advancement of RA in addition to just relieving symptoms. The cardiovascular system also benefits from the anti-inflammatory qualities, which may lower the risk of cardiovascular diseases, which is frequently higher in RA patients. These benefits go beyond joint health.

Given the role that omega-3 fatty acids play in the management of RA, it is imperative to include sources of these vital nutrients in one's daily diet. People with RA can take advantage of the anti-inflammatory properties of omega-3 fatty acids to support their overall joint health, whether by eating fish regularly or by including plant-based options like hemp and chia seeds.

The Function of Antioxidants in Combined Protection

A rheumatoid arthritis diet must include antioxidants because they are vital in shielding joints from inflammation and oxidative stress. When healthy tissues are mistakenly attacked by the immune system in RA, highly reactive molecules known as free radicals are released, which can cause cell damage, inflammation, and joint degradation.

Antioxidants, which are abundant in fruits and vegetables, play a crucial role in reducing the overall oxidative burden on the body by neutralizing free radicals. Selenium, beta-carotene, and vitamins C and E are important antioxidants that have been linked to joint protection in RA patients. These antioxidants are abundant in citrus fruits, berries, nuts, and spinach.

Antioxidants not only directly scavenge free radicals but also have anti-inflammatory qualities. Antioxidants help to manage RA symptoms overall by lowering inflammation and regulating immune responses. Furthermore, by enhancing the anti-inflammatory properties of drugs, they might enhance the efficacy of traditional RA therapies.

To guarantee that they consume enough antioxidants, people with RA must include a wide variety of vibrant fruits and vegetables in their diet. Eating by the colors of the rainbow offers a range of antioxidants and tastes as well as protection for joints and general health.

<u>Minerals and Vitamins for the Treatment of Rheumatoid Arthritis</u>

Beyond just treating the symptoms, rheumatoid arthritis management involves adding certain vitamins and minerals that are essential for maintaining the immune system and joint health. For example, vitamin D plays a critical role in calcium absorption and bone health. This is especially true for people with RA, who may be more susceptible to osteoporosis as a result of inflammation and medication use.

Furthermore, the synthesis of collagen, a protein that makes up ligaments, tendons, and joints, depends on vitamin C. Consuming foods high in vitamin C, such as bell peppers, strawberries, and citrus fruits, helps to maintain the structure and function of joints.

Magnesium and calcium are two minerals that cooperate to support healthy bones and muscles. For people with RA, it is especially important to make sure they are getting enough of these minerals because joint pain and inflammation can affect bone density and muscle strength. Good dietary sources of calcium and magnesium include dairy products, nuts, and leafy greens.

Furthermore, due to their critical roles in immune function, zinc and selenium deficiencies have been linked to an increased risk of infection, which may be concerning for people with RA whose immune systems are already compromised. Including foods high in selenium, like Brazil nuts, and foods high in zinc, like meat, beans, and seeds, can help support the immune system.

In summary, a variety of nutrient-dense foods included in a well-balanced diet are essential for managing rheumatoid arthritis. In addition to meeting nutritional needs, a diet rich in omega-3 fatty acids, antioxidants, vitamins, and minerals promotes joint health, lowers inflammation, and improves general well-being in people with RA.

CHAPTER FOUR

FOODS YOU SHOULD EAT IF YOU HAVE RHEUMATOID ARTHRITIS

Fish and Foods High in Omega-3

Because of their anti-inflammatory qualities, fish and foods high in omega-3 fatty acids are essential components of a diet for rheumatoid arthritis (RA). It has been demonstrated that omega-3 fatty acids, in particular, eicosapentaenoic acid (EPA) and docosahexaenoic acid (DHA), which are present in fatty fish like salmon, mackerel, and sardines, can help lower inflammation and relieve RA symptoms. These vital fatty acids suppress the immune system and prevent the synthesis of inflammatory chemicals.

Additionally, pro-resolving lipid mediators (SPMs), which actively reduce inflammation and support tissue repair, are produced in part by omega-3 fatty acids. Incorporating fish into the diet offers a nutrient-rich package that includes protein, vitamin D, and selenium, all of which are critical for the general health of joints in addition to a direct supply of these advantageous fatty acids.

Fish must be a regular part of the diet for people suffering from RA. Fish oil capsules or other omega-3 supplements may be an option if eating fish is difficult. However, to guarantee the right dosage and safety, speaking with a healthcare provider before beginning any supplement regimen is advised.

Vibrantly colored fruits and veggies

A diet rich in color-rich fruits and vegetables is essential for people with rheumatoid arthritis because it offers a plethora of antioxidants, vitamins, and minerals. Colorful pigments found in fruits and vegetables, like the carotenoids in bell peppers and carrots, and the flavonoids in citrus fruits and berries, have strong anti-inflammatory effects. These substances aid in the fight against oxidative stress, which is frequently more severe in RA patients.

Fruits and vegetables are rich in fiber, which supports gut health and may have unintentional anti-inflammatory effects, in addition to antioxidants. It is becoming more widely acknowledged that controlling inflammatory diseases, such as rheumatoid arthritis, requires a healthy gut microbiome. A wide spectrum of nutrients, such as vitamin C, vitamin K, and folate, which are critical for joint health and general well-being, are ensured by eating a variety of fruits and vegetables.

Variety is key because different fruits and vegetables offer special phytonutrients that have different anti-inflammatory and immune-modulating properties. Using a variety of colors on the plate can be a useful way to take advantage of all the health advantages that these plant-based foods have to offer.

Fiber and Whole Grains

In a diet for rheumatoid arthritis, whole grains and dietary fiber are important because they support gut health in general and may have an impact on inflammatory processes. Complex carbohydrates found in whole grains, like brown rice, quinoa, and whole wheat, release energy gradually and contribute to stable blood sugar levels.

A healthy gut microbiome is supported by fiber, which is abundant in whole grains, legumes, fruits, and vegetables. Reducing inflammation is linked to a balanced and diverse microbiome, which is important for controlling the symptoms of rheumatoid arthritis. Furthermore, soluble fiber in particular has been connected to decreased levels of the inflammatory marker C-reactive protein (CRP).

To optimize their nutrient intake, people with RA are advised to choose whole grains over refined grains. Choosing whole wheat pasta, brown rice, and whole grain bread are examples of this. Including a range of these grains in the diet improves long-term joint health and increases nutritional diversity.

Trimmed Meats and Plant-Based Substitutes

The selection of proteins is critical in a diet for rheumatoid arthritis, and lean protein sources are essential for reducing inflammation and enhancing joint health. Lean meats are high in quality protein without having the excess saturated fats of fattier cuts of meat. Examples of lean meats include poultry, lean cuts of beef, and lean pork. Protein is necessary for the upkeep of muscles, and people with RA must sustain joint function by keeping their muscles strong.

If a plant-based diet is preferred, many plant-based protein substitutes can be included in the diet. In addition to providing high-quality plant-based proteins, legumes, tofu, tempeh, and edamame also provide a range of vital nutrients and fiber.

For a complete intake of essential amino acids, it's critical to find a balance and combine both plant- and animal-based proteins. Furthermore, incorporating omega-3 fatty acid sources like flaxseeds and chia seeds into plant-based meals can intensify their anti-inflammatory qualities.

People with rheumatoid arthritis can actively manage inflammation and joint symptoms while also supporting their overall health and well-being by focusing on lean proteins and plant-based alternatives.

CHAPTER FIVE

THE EFFECTS OF DAIRY AND GLUTEN

Gluten Intolerance in Rheumatoid Arthritis Patients

In the context of rheumatoid arthritis (RA), gluten sensitivity has drawn more attention as researchers explore the complex relationship between dietary factors and autoimmune diseases. Wheat, barley, and rye all contain the protein gluten, which some people with RA may be more sensitive to. Although non-celiac gluten sensitivity (NCGS) is not the same as celiac disease, it is a known gluten-related condition that may also exacerbate RA symptoms.

Studies have indicated that gluten sensitivity could be linked to systemic inflammation, which is a defining feature of RA. Gluten consumption may set off an immunological reaction in those who are susceptible, resulting in the release of inflammatory cytokines and the activation of immune cells. Patients with RA may experience worsening joint inflammation as a result of this inflammatory cascade. Furthermore, gluten sensitivity must be taken into account when creating a rheumatoid arthritis diet because it may not only exacerbate symptoms but also slow the disease's progression.

A gluten-free diet has emerged as a key component in the management of RA in people with gluten sensitivity. Although removing gluten-containing grains from one's diet won't cure RA, it may lessen symptoms and enhance the lives of those who are impacted. Collaborating closely with healthcare professionals and nutritionists is crucial for patients with RA, as it guarantees a well-rounded and sufficient gluten-free diet tailored to their requirements.

Milk and Inflammation: Essential Information

In light of rheumatoid arthritis, the connection between dairy consumption and inflammation has drawn attention. Proteins found in dairy products like milk and cheese can stimulate the immune system and possibly cause inflammation. Examining the effects of dairy on inflammatory pathways is critical because controlling inflammation is a key component of treatment for people with RA.

Casein is a milk protein that plays a major role in inflammation related to dairy products. Some people may have an intolerance to casein, which triggers an immunological reaction and causes the release of substances that promote inflammation. Furthermore, some dairy products' saturated fats may increase inflammation and exacerbate RA symptoms in certain people. According to studies, eating a diet high in saturated fats may cause an imbalance in the body's inflammatory response, which could make RA worse.

Because of this, a lot of people with RA think about switching to a low- or no-dairy diet to control inflammation and reduce symptoms. This entails switching out conventional dairy products with plant-based milk, yogurt, and cheese as substitutes. But it's important to make sure these substitutes are sufficiently nourished and offer vital elements like calcium and vitamin D, which are frequently found in large amounts in dairy products.

Investigating Dairy-Free and Gluten-Free Substitutions

While following a gluten- and dairy-free diet can be difficult, researching substitutes is crucial for rheumatoid arthritis sufferers who want to reduce their symptoms. Using gluten-free substitutes for traditional grains often entails switching to rice, quinoa, and gluten-free oats. Not only do these grains make good substitutes, but they also add extra nutrients to the diet that promote general health.

In a similar vein, dairy-free substitutes have grown in acceptance, providing people with RA with a variety of choices without sacrificing nutritional content. Rich in vitamins and minerals, plant-based milk made from almonds, soy, or oats offers a lactose-free substitute.

For individuals who want to manage their rheumatoid arthritis symptoms while still maintaining a varied and enjoyable diet, non-dairy yogurts and cheeses made from coconut, almond, or cashews provide satisfying options.

When looking for gluten- and dairy-free substitutes, RA sufferers need to continue to pay attention to nutritional balance.

It can be helpful to collaborate with nutritionists and healthcare providers to create a personalized diet plan that not only takes into account dietary restrictions but also guarantees the consumption of vital nutrients for optimum health.

People with rheumatoid arthritis can make educated dietary decisions to better manage their illness and enhance their general well-being by investigating these options.

CHAPTER SIX

MANAGING WEIGHT FOR JOINT HEALTH

The Relationship Between Weight and Rheumatoid Arthritis

Sustaining a healthy weight is essential for the management of rheumatoid arthritis (RA) since being overweight can worsen the symptoms and course of this autoimmune disease. The hallmark of rheumatoid arthritis is joint inflammation, which causes discomfort, edema, and stiffness.

Being overweight puts extra strain on the joints, especially the spine, hips, and knees, making RA patients feel more uncomfortable. Additionally, inflammatory chemicals called cytokines are produced by adipose tissue, and these substances can exacerbate the inflammatory response in the joints. Because of this, people with RA frequently discover that reaching and keeping an ideal weight is essential to the overall management of their illness.

Studies have consistently demonstrated a link between obesity and a higher chance of rheumatoid arthritis. Adipokines are signaling molecules secreted by adipose tissue that are involved in inflammation and may cause or exacerbate symptoms of RA.

Furthermore, elevated levels of C-reactive protein (CRP), a biomarker of inflammation in the body, are linked to obesity. Rheumatoid arthritis patients frequently have elevated CRP levels, and being overweight can exacerbate this inflammatory reaction.

Recognizing the complex relationship between weight and RA highlights the significance of weight control as a cornerstone of the comprehensive treatment strategy.

Techniques for Maintaining a Healthful Weight

In the context of rheumatoid arthritis, effective weight control is a multimodal strategy that incorporates dietary adjustments, physical activity, and lifestyle alterations. Eating a diet high in fruits, vegetables, whole grains, and lean proteins—which are known to reduce inflammation—can aid in weight loss. It has been demonstrated that consuming omega-3 fatty acids, which are present in fish oil and flaxseeds, has anti-inflammatory properties that may help reduce the symptoms of RA and support weight management.

Another crucial component of weight management for people with rheumatoid arthritis is portion control. Overeating can be avoided and metabolism can be regulated by eating smaller, more frequent meals. Furthermore, it's critical to maintain proper hydration because, on occasion, dehydration might be mistaken for hunger, which can result in unneeded calorie intake. Consulting with a qualified dietitian can offer tailored nutritional advice, ensuring that dietary selections meet the unique requirements of people with RA as well as weight management objectives.

Exercise's Impact on Joint Health and Weight Control

The key to controlling weight and maintaining joint health in those with rheumatoid arthritis is regular exercise. Low-impact exercises that don't overly strain the joints, like walking, cycling, or swimming, can help reduce body fat, strengthen the heart, and preserve joint flexibility. Exercises for strengthening the muscles around injured joints help reduce the stress that extra body weight places on these delicate areas by adding stability and support.

In addition, exercise is essential for battling the exhaustion that rheumatoid arthritis frequently causes. Even though exhaustion can make exercising appear intimidating, a well-thought-out fitness regimen can increase energy and improve one's general sense of well-being. The best exercises for controlling weight and rheumatoid arthritis symptoms can be chosen by customizing workout regimens to each person's ability and seeking advice from medical specialists or physical therapists. To summarize, a comprehensive strategy that includes portion management, food adjustments, and consistent exercise is necessary for rheumatoid arthritis patients who want to properly manage their weight and support joint health.

CHAPTER SEVEN

USEFUL ADVICE FOR DAILY EATING

Organizing Your Meals for Rheumatoid Arthritis

When it comes to maintaining a healthy, well-balanced diet and controlling rheumatoid arthritis (RA), meal planning is essential. It is imperative to prioritize the consumption of foods that have anti-inflammatory qualities to mitigate symptoms related to RA.

Inflammation is reduced by a Mediterranean-style diet high in fruits, vegetables, whole grains, and healthy fats. Including a choice of vibrant fruits and vegetables guarantees a varied spectrum of antioxidants, vitamins, and minerals that are good for joint health.

Adding omega-3 fatty acids—which are present in walnuts, flaxseeds, and fatty seafood like salmon—is also advised. These good fats can help to improve joint function and have anti-inflammatory qualities. Lean protein sources like chicken, beans, and tofu also help maintain muscle health and supply essential nutrients without aggravating inflammation. Brown rice and quinoa are examples of whole grains that can be great providers of fiber and support digestive health in general.

Those who have RA can think about eating smaller, more frequent meals throughout the day to keep their blood sugar levels consistent. In addition to offering a consistent supply of nutrients to promote joint function, this can assist in avoiding energy dumps. Finally, drinking plenty of water throughout the day is necessary for maintaining proper hydration, which is important for general health and can help reduce inflammation.

Methods of Cooking to Preserve Maximum Nutrient Content

The methods of cooking used to prepare food for people with rheumatoid arthritis can have a big impact on the food's nutritional value and general health benefits. The best cooking techniques are steaming, sautéing, and grilling since they enable fruits and vegetables to keep as much of their nutrients as possible. Vegetables cooked gently (without high temperatures) and with the vitamins and minerals preserved by steaming have a lower chance of losing nutrients.

Healthy oils, like olive oil, improve the flavor and improve the absorption of fat-soluble vitamins when sautéed. Grilling is another technique that provides a unique taste to food without compromising its nutritious content. However, it's vital to prevent charring or overcooking, as this might introduce toxic compounds and nullify the advantages of the chosen ingredients.

When preparing meats, it's preferable to choose lean cuts and apply cooking methods that maintain moisture, such as baking or slow cooking. These approaches assist in preserving the protein content while limiting the development of potentially inflammatory chemicals associated with high-heat cooking.

Dining Out and Making Informed Choices

Maintaining a rheumatoid arthritis-friendly diet extends beyond home-cooked meals, and making informed choices when dining out is equally vital. When reading a menu, picking dishes containing a range of colorful veggies, lean proteins, and whole grains is suggested. Grilled or steamed selections are frequently healthier choices compared to fried or excessively processed alternatives.

Communication with restaurant workers is crucial. It's appropriate to ask about cooking methods, ingredients, and potential alternatives to tailor a meal to dietary demands.

Many places are accommodative and willing to adapt dishes to match individual requests.

Choosing carefully from the menu also requires being mindful of quantity proportions. RA sufferers may benefit from smaller, more frequent meals, so choosing appetizers or half servings can be a strategic approach. Additionally, avoiding excessive salt and opting for foods with herbs and spices for flavor can help to a better dining experience.

Being proactive about dietary choices while dining out helps individuals with rheumatoid arthritis to enjoy meals outside the home without compromising their nutritional goals.

CHAPTER EIGHT

SUPPLEMENTS AND THEIR ROLE

Overview of Dietary Supplements

Dietary supplements play a crucial part in managing rheumatoid arthritis (RA), allowing consumers an extra approach to reduce symptoms and improve overall joint health. While they can not replace conventional medical treatments, supplements can complement them by addressing nutritional deficiencies and supporting the body's natural activities. Understanding the impact of these supplements in the context of an RA diet is vital for those seeking comprehensive ways to control their condition.

One of the essential components in the supplement regimen for RA is omega-3 fatty acids. Found in fish oil and flaxseed oil, these essential fatty acids have anti-inflammatory qualities that may help relieve joint discomfort and stiffness. Additionally, vitamin D is typically advised as it plays a key role in bone health, a worry for patients with RA who may be at an increased risk of osteoporosis. The immune-modulating effects of probiotics have also received interest, as they may help maintain a balanced gut flora, impacting the overall inflammatory response in the body.

Another important supplement is turmeric, which contains curcumin, which has anti-inflammatory and antioxidant characteristics. Some studies suggest that curcumin may help relieve joint discomfort and morning stiffness in patients with RA. Furthermore, glucosamine and chondroitin, natural components of cartilage, are typically included in supplement programs for RA. While research results are inconsistent, some individuals report improvements in joint pain and function with these supplements.

It is necessary to approach supplementing with caution, considering potential interactions with drugs and individual variances in response. Striking a balance between receiving vital nutrients and avoiding excessive amounts is critical to maintaining the safety and efficacy of dietary supplements in the context of RA therapy.

Common Supplements for Rheumatoid Arthritis

In the domain of rheumatoid arthritis (RA) management, various supplements have garnered recognition for their potential to ease symptoms and enhance overall joint health. Fish oil, rich in omega-3 fatty acids, stands out as a widespread and well-researched supplement. The anti-inflammatory characteristics of omega-3s have been associated with reduced joint discomfort and stiffness in persons with RA. Incorporating fish oil into the diet or opting for supplements might be a beneficial complement for those seeking natural ways to treat their disease.

Vitamin D is another highly suggested vitamin for patients with RA. Beyond its vital role in bone health, vitamin D has immunomodulatory properties that may aid patients with autoimmune disorders like RA. Many persons with RA have low levels of vitamin D, and supplementation might help rectify this deficit, thereby promoting general well-being.

Turmeric, notably its main ingredient curcumin, has attracted attention for its anti-inflammatory and antioxidant qualities. Some studies suggest that curcumin may help relieve joint discomfort and morning stiffness in patients with RA. While further research is needed, turmeric pills or integrating this spice into dishes may offer a tasty and perhaps beneficial component to an RA diet.

Glucosamine and chondroitin, natural components of cartilage, are routinely included in supplement programs for RA. Despite inconsistent research results, some individuals claim improvements in joint pain and function with these substances. It's important to remember that individual reactions might vary, and speaking with a healthcare practitioner is crucial before including these supplements in an RA management regimen.

As with any therapy method, patients with RA must discuss supplement use with their healthcare provider. This ensures that supplements correspond with their overall treatment plan and do not interfere with prescribed drugs.

Healthcare specialists can provide individualized counsel based on an individual's specific health situation, helping to enhance the possible advantages of supplements while reducing any hazards.

Consultation with Healthcare Professionals

When selecting a rheumatoid arthritis (RA) diet that incorporates dietary supplements, contact with healthcare providers is crucial. While supplements can offer additional support, they are not a substitute for established medical therapies. Engaging with healthcare providers ensures a holistic and coordinated strategy for controlling RA, taking into account individual health conditions, medications, and potential interactions.

Before adopting any supplements into an RA management regimen, consumers should check with their rheumatologist or primary care physician. These healthcare professionals can examine the unique needs of the individual, including aspects such as the severity of RA, overall health, and any existing nutritional deficits. This tailored approach helps adjust the supplement regimen to address individual needs and promote overall health.

Healthcare experts play a critical role in guiding individuals through the complexity of supplement use, giving evidence-based advice, and monitoring for any potential adverse effects or interactions. They can offer insights into the latest study findings and assist individuals in making informed selections about the best appropriate supplements for their condition.

Additionally, healthcare experts can review the general dietary patterns of persons with RA, ensuring that nutritional demands are satisfied through a balanced and well-rounded diet. This includes correcting any shortages in vitamins and minerals, which can dramatically impair joint health and overall well-being.

Regular follow-ups with healthcare professionals are required to check the effectiveness of the supplement regimen and make any necessary modifications. They can also track changes in RA symptoms, ensuring that the treatment regimen remains matched with the individual's growing health state.

In conclusion, the collaboration between individuals with RA and their healthcare experts is vital for the safe and effective integration of dietary supplements into an RA management strategy. This relationship ensures that supplement use is evidence-based, customized to individual needs, and part of a complete approach to managing rheumatoid arthritis.

CHAPTER NINE

LIFESTYLE FACTORS AND RHEUMATOID ARTHRITIS

<u>Stress Management Techniques in the Context of Rheumatoid Arthritis Diet</u>

Stress, both physical and emotional, has been found as a crucial factor in determining the severity of rheumatoid arthritis (RA). In the context of an RA diet, stress management techniques play a significant role in reducing symptoms and boosting general well-being. Chronic stress can aggravate inflammation, a hallmark of RA, and provoke flare-ups. Therefore, integrating appropriate stress management measures is crucial for patients with RA.

One essential stress management strategy is mindfulness meditation. This technique enables individuals to focus on the present moment, generating a sense of serenity and decreasing the impact of stress on the body. Mindful eating, an outgrowth of mindfulness, is particularly useful for people following an RA diet. It involves paying close attention to food choices, relishing each meal, and being attentive to how different foods influence the body. This not only benefits stress reduction but also promotes healthy eating habits.

Another valuable stress management strategy is regular physical activity. Engaging in exercises such as yoga or tai chi not only aids in preserving joint flexibility but also works as a strong stress reliever. Exercise causes the release of endorphins, the body's natural mood boosters, contributing to an improved emotional state. It is vital, however, to adjust exercise programs to individual capacities, recognizing the special obstacles offered by RA.

Counseling and therapy are additional possibilities for stress management. Living with a chronic condition like RA can be emotionally exhausting, and seeking professional support can provide coping mechanisms and emotional resilience. Incorporating such mental health methods into the entire approach to RA, including nutritional concerns, gives a comprehensive framework for controlling the condition.

The Importance of Adequate Sleep in the Context of Rheumatoid Arthritis Diet

Adequate and quality sleep is a cornerstone of overall health, and its relevance becomes even more obvious in the context of rheumatoid arthritis (RA). Sleep plays a key part in the body's ability to repair and regenerate, and for those with RA, it directly affects the intensity of symptoms and the body's inflammatory response.

In the domain of an RA diet, promoting proper sleep hygiene is crucial. Establishing a consistent sleep schedule, creating a comfortable sleep environment, and minimizing stimulants, particularly close to bedtime, are key factors. Sleep difficulties are frequent among patients with RA, and managing these disruptions becomes crucial to the overall care of the condition.

Moreover, the association between poor sleep and heightened pain sensitivity in RA highlights the significance of treating sleep as part of the nutritional plan. Chronic sleep deprivation can contribute to increased pain perception and worsen joint stiffness, both of which are important issues for patients with RA. Thus, an RA diet should not only focus on nutritional components but also emphasize the formation of conducive conditions for peaceful and restorative sleep.

Incorporating relaxation techniques, such as mild stretching or breathing exercises, before bedtime can further boost sleep quality. Additionally, technology usage, particularly screen time before sleep, should be restricted, as the blue light released can interfere with the body's natural sleep-wake cycle.

Balancing Physical Activity for Joint Health in the Context of Rheumatoid Arthritis Diet

Balancing physical activity is a vital component of controlling rheumatoid arthritis (RA), especially when considering its impact on joint health within the framework of an RA diet. Exercise is generally viewed as a double-edged sword for those with RA — it is necessary for maintaining joint function and overall well-being, yet the improper method can exacerbate symptoms. Striking the appropriate balance is crucial.

Low-impact workouts, such as swimming or walking, are particularly good for patients with RA. These workouts provide circulatory advantages without putting excessive strain on the joints. When paired with an RA diet rich in anti-inflammatory foods, the synergy can contribute to a complete strategy for managing the condition.

However, it is vital to customize physical activity to individual capacities and illness development. Consulting with a healthcare expert or a physical therapist is advisable to design a specific workout regimen. Incorporating joint-friendly activities into everyday routines, such as range-of-motion exercises and strength training, can aid in maintaining flexibility and muscle strength without exerting undue stress on the joints.

Moreover, pacing oneself during physical activities is vital. Overexertion can contribute to increased inflammation and exhaustion, common issues for patients with RA. Integrating moments of rest and recovery into a workout regimen is as crucial as the activity itself. This balanced approach coincides with the goals of an RA diet, stressing general health and wellness while addressing the unique needs of joint health.

In conclusion, achieving harmony between physical activity and dietary concerns is vital for persons with RA. The primary goal is to develop a lifestyle that supports joint health, mitigates inflammation, and enhances overall quality of life.

CHAPTER TEN

PERSONALIZED APPROACHES TO DIET

Understanding Individual Triggers

Rheumatoid arthritis (RA) is a chronic inflammatory illness that mostly affects the joints. While there is no proven treatment for RA, tailored approaches to food have received interest as a strategy to control symptoms and enhance general well-being. Understanding individual triggers is a vital component of creating a nutrition plan for patients with rheumatoid arthritis. Each person may react differently to certain meals, and identifying certain triggers can aid in regulating inflammation and decreasing discomfort.

The first step in determining individual triggers includes realizing that rheumatoid arthritis is an autoimmune condition where the immune system wrongly targets the joints. Certain foods may promote inflammation and stimulate immunological responses, leading to greater joint pain and stiffness. Common causes include processed foods, heavy consumption of red meat, and foods high in refined carbohydrates. However, the influence of these triggers can differ from person to person.

To find particular triggers, persons with rheumatoid arthritis often complete an elimination diet. This entails temporarily removing suspected trigger foods and then gradually returning them while monitoring for any adverse effects. Additionally, advanced testing methods, such as food sensitivity testing, may provide insights into specific foods that could be contributing to inflammation. This individualized method helps patients to discover and remove foods that may worsen their rheumatoid arthritis symptoms.

Keeping a Food Diary for Self-Discovery

Maintaining a food diary is a useful tool in the customized control of rheumatoid arthritis through diet. A food diary allows individuals to document their daily food intake, evaluate symptoms, and find trends or correlations between diet and arthritis flare-ups. This self-discovery approach helps individuals make informed decisions about their dietary choices based on their unique sensitivities to different foods.

In the food diary, users note not only what they eat but also the timing of meals, portion quantities, and any obvious symptoms or changes in arthritic symptoms. This diligent tracking helps establish linkages between specific foods and the worsening of rheumatoid arthritis symptoms. It also provides vital information for healthcare experts when designing tailored food recommendations.

A food diary acts as a dynamic tool for individuals to take charge of their rheumatoid arthritis management. By spotting patterns over time, individuals can make proactive alterations to their diets, removing potential triggers and adopting items that improve joint health. This individualized and self-directed approach can lead to a greater knowledge of the intricate interaction between nutrition and rheumatoid arthritis, permitting more effective symptom management.

Seeking Professional Guidance for Personalized Plans

While self-discovery through a food diary is helpful, getting professional guidance is a critical step in building highly tailored diet programs for rheumatoid arthritis. Healthcare specialists, such as registered dietitians or nutritionists with expertise in autoimmune disorders, can offer individualized guidance based on an individual's specific health profile, dietary preferences, and lifestyle.

These professionals can conduct a full examination, taking into consideration aspects such as the severity of rheumatoid arthritis, overall health, and any other medical disorders. A personalized diet plan may incorporate recommendations for anti-inflammatory foods, optimal portion sizes, and specific nutrients that support joint health.

Moreover, doctors can educate clients on boosting their diets with key nutrients like omega-3 fatty acids, recognized for their anti-inflammatory qualities.

Professional advice is particularly crucial in ensuring that patients with rheumatoid arthritis receive appropriate nutrition while avoiding harmful triggers. Registered dietitians can assist individuals in managing difficult dietary restrictions and establishing balanced meal plans that satisfy their nutritional needs.

This collaborative approach guarantees that tailored food programs match with overall health goals and contribute to the effective management of rheumatoid arthritis symptoms.

CHAPTER ELEVEN

OVERCOMING CHALLENGES AND STAYING MOTIVATED

Addressing Common Hurdles in Adhering to the Diet

One of the biggest obstacles individuals confront when adopting a rheumatoid arthritis (RA) diet is the requirement for considerable lifestyle modifications. The dietary alterations suggested for controlling RA frequently involve avoiding particular foods that may promote inflammation and embracing a more anti-inflammatory and nutrient-rich eating plan.

Transitioning to this new way of eating can be frightening, especially if it entails changing long-established habits. Moreover, external circumstances such as social events and restaurant visits may provide difficulties, making it challenging to stick closely to the prescribed diet.

To overcome these barriers, it is necessary to plan and prepare meals in advance, explain dietary preferences to friends and family, and discover inventive methods to enjoy social gatherings without breaching the dietary guidelines.

Additionally, working together with a healthcare expert or nutritionist can provide personalized assistance and practical techniques for overcoming these frequent difficulties.

<u>Staying Positive and Focused on Long-Term Health</u>

Maintaining a positive outlook is key to effectively navigating the hurdles of an RA diet. Chronic illnesses like rheumatoid arthritis can impact multiple elements of everyday living, and dietary adjustments are often just one part of a holistic care approach. It's crucial to regard the diet not as a limiting burden but as a proactive move towards greater health and symptom control. Setting realistic objectives and milestones, appreciating little triumphs, and recognizing the positive influence of dietary changes on overall well-being can lead to a more optimistic approach. Additionally, adopting mindfulness and stress-reduction practices can assist in managing the emotional components of living with a chronic disease. By concentrating on the long-term health benefits and keeping a resilient attitude, individuals can better cope with the challenges and stay motivated to adhere to the RA diet over time.

Connecting with Supportive Communities

Building a network of support is vital for persons navigating the challenges of an RA diet. Connecting with individuals who share similar experiences can bring a sense of solidarity and understanding. Online forums, support groups, and social media communities dedicated to rheumatoid arthritis can be great resources for exchanging practical information, sharing success stories, and seeking guidance on overcoming specific issues connected to the diet. Engaging with healthcare specialists, particularly rheumatologists, nutritionists, and dietitians, can also offer assistance and encouragement. Additionally, integrating friends and family in the journey helps establish a supportive environment at home, ensuring that those close to the individual with RA are aware of and attentive to the dietary requirements. By creating relationships within the RA community and beyond, individuals can find encouragement, inspiration, and a shared sense of purpose in adhering to the suggested diet for rheumatoid arthritis.

CHAPTER TWELVE

BEYOND DIET: COMPREHENSIVE RHEUMATOID ARTHRITIS MANAGEMENT

Medication and Treatment Options

In the field of Rheumatoid Arthritis (RA) management, a multidisciplinary strategy is typically needed to address the intricacies of the condition. Medications have a vital role in easing symptoms, slowing down the progression of the disease, and enhancing the overall quality of life for patients with RA. Nonsteroidal anti-inflammatory medications (NSAIDs) are routinely applied to control pain and inflammation. These drugs, such as ibuprofen and naproxen, function by lowering the formation of prostaglandins, molecules that contribute to inflammation.

Another class of drugs used in RA treatment are Disease-Modifying Antirheumatic Drugs (DMARDs), which target the immune system to change its response. Conventional DMARDs like methotrexate and newer biological DMARDs like adalimumab have proved efficacy in slowing down joint deterioration and enhancing function. Corticosteroids, such as prednisone, may be administered to ease severe symptoms in the short term. However, their long-term use is frequently limited due to probable negative effects.

In some circumstances, healthcare practitioners may recommend a combination of these medications to obtain optimal results. The choice of treatment relies on the severity of the ailment, the patient's overall health, and any adverse effects. Regular monitoring and modifications to the treatment plan are common practices to achieve the most effective and well-tolerated therapy.

Beyond pharmaceutical therapies, surgical procedures may be considered for people with extensive joint degeneration. Joint replacement surgery, particularly for knees and hips, can dramatically boost mobility and alleviate discomfort. However, these operations are normally reserved for cases where conservative methods have proven ineffective.

Collaborating with Healthcare Providers

The collaborative cooperation between individuals with RA and their healthcare professionals is crucial to attaining good outcomes in controlling the condition. RA is a chronic condition that demands continual communication and cooperation between patients and healthcare professionals.

Regular appointments and open communication enable healthcare practitioners to assess disease activity, monitor drug efficacy, and address any emergent issues.

Patients are urged to actively participate in their care by providing thorough information about their symptoms, medication adherence, and overall well-being. This proactive involvement helps healthcare providers to adjust treatment approaches to the particular needs of each patient. Furthermore, routine laboratory testing and imaging examinations may be performed to evaluate disease development and the impact of treatment.

Patient education is an important component of collaborative care, helping individuals to understand their condition and make educated decisions about their health. This involves teaching patients about the potential negative effects of drugs, lifestyle adjustments, and the significance of regular exercise. Additionally, healthcare experts may offer help in managing stress, as stress can increase RA symptoms.

A multidisciplinary approach to care, combining rheumatologists, physical therapists, occupational therapists, and other professionals, can provide a comprehensive support system. This collaborative network guarantees that all elements of RA, including physical, emotional, and functional well-being, are addressed holistically.

Holistic Approaches to Enhance Overall Well-Being

While drugs and medical interventions are key components of RA management, a holistic strategy that involves lifestyle adjustments and self-care measures is equally vital. Holistic approaches attempt to increase total well-being by addressing the physical, emotional, and social components of life.

Diet plays a crucial part in the comprehensive management of RA. Certain foods, such as those high in omega-3 fatty acids (found in fish), antioxidants (found in fruits and vegetables), and anti-inflammatory characteristics (found in turmeric and ginger), may help ease symptoms. Conversely, some persons with RA may benefit from avoiding specific foods that could increase inflammation.

Regular physical activity is another cornerstone of a comprehensive approach. Exercise helps maintain joint flexibility, build muscles, and enhance overall cardiovascular health. Tailored exercise programs, established in consultation with healthcare practitioners and physical therapists, can be important in controlling RA symptoms.

Stress management strategies, such as mindfulness meditation, deep breathing exercises, and yoga, can contribute to emotional well-being. Chronic stress has been related to increasing RA symptoms, and implementing stress-reducing activities into daily life can have positive impacts on both mental and physical health.

Adequate sleep is vital for patients with RA, as exhaustion is a common symptom of the condition. Establishing a regular sleep regimen, providing a comfortable sleep environment, and addressing any underlying sleep issues can greatly enhance energy levels and general quality of life.

Social support and establishing a strong support network are crucial components of holistic RA care. Connecting with others who understand the hardships of living with RA can provide emotional support and practical ideas. Online and in-person support groups provide a forum for people to exchange helpful information, coping mechanisms, and personal experiences.

In summary, a holistic strategy to improve general well-being, cooperation with healthcare practitioners, and pharmaceutical and therapy alternatives are all part of a comprehensive approach to managing rheumatoid arthritis. Individuals suffering from RA can aim for enhanced functional ability, better quality of life, and better symptom control by incorporating these components into a customized care plan.

30 DAY MEAL PLAN

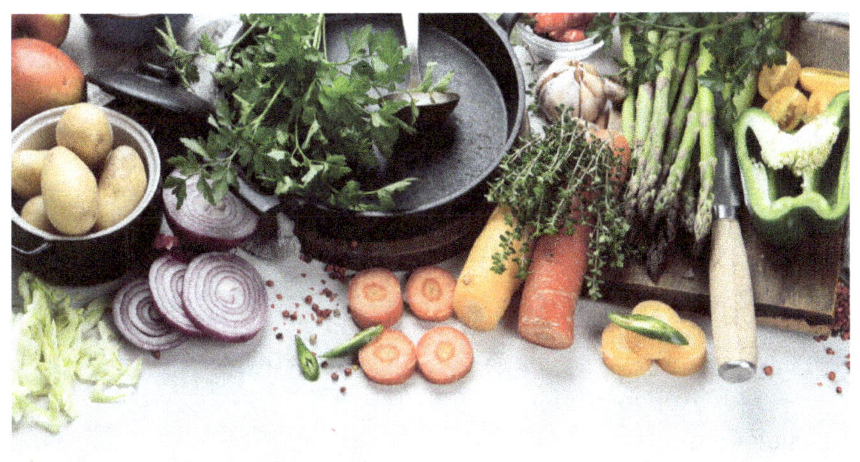

This meal plan incorporates anti-inflammatory ingredients that may help reduce symptoms associated with Rheumatoid Arthritis. Adjustments can be made according to individual preferences and dietary restrictions.

Day 1

Breakfast: Turmeric Oatmeal

Ingredients:

- 1/2 cup rolled oats

- 1 cup water or almond milk

- 1/2 teaspoon turmeric powder

- 1/4 teaspoon ground cinnamon

- 1 tablespoon honey or maple syrup (optional)

- 1/4 cup blueberries

- 1 tablespoon chopped walnuts

Cooking Directions:

1. In a saucepan, bring water or almond milk to a boil.

2. Stir in rolled oats, turmeric, and cinnamon.

3. Reduce heat to low and simmer for 5-7 minutes, stirring occasionally.

4. Once cooked, remove from heat and sweeten with honey or maple syrup if desired.

5. Top with blueberries and chopped walnuts before serving.

Prep Time: 10 minutes

Servings: 1

Lunch: Anti-Inflammatory Chickpea Salad

Ingredients:

- 1 cup canned chickpeas, drained and rinsed

- 1/2 cucumber, diced

- 1/2 cup cherry tomatoes, halved

- 1/4 cup diced red onion

- 2 tablespoons chopped fresh parsley

- 1 tablespoon extra virgin olive oil

- 1 tablespoon lemon juice

- Salt and pepper to taste

Assembly:

1. In a bowl, combine chickpeas, cucumber, cherry tomatoes, red onion, and parsley.

2. Drizzle with olive oil and lemon juice.

3. Season with salt and pepper, then toss to coat.

4. Serve chilled or at room temperature.

Prep Time: 10 minutes

Servings: 2

Dinner: Ginger-Garlic Salmon with Quinoa and Steamed Broccoli

Ingredients:

- 2 salmon fillets

- 1 teaspoon grated ginger

- 2 cloves garlic, minced

- 1 tablespoon soy sauce (low-sodium)

- 1 tablespoon honey

- 1 tablespoon olive oil

- 1 cup cooked quinoa

- 2 cups steamed broccoli

Cooking Directions:

1. Preheat oven to 375°F (190°C).

2. In a small bowl, mix grated ginger, minced garlic, soy sauce, honey, and olive oil.

3. Place salmon fillets on a baking sheet lined with parchment paper.

4. Brush the ginger-garlic mixture over the salmon.

5. Bake for 12-15 minutes or until salmon is cooked through.

6. Serve salmon with cooked quinoa and steamed broccoli.

Prep Time: 15 minutes

Cook Time: 15 minutes

Servings: 2

Snack: Carrot Sticks with Hummus

Ingredients:

- 2 carrots, cut into sticks

- 1/4 cup hummus

Assembly:

1. Dip carrot sticks into hummus and enjoy.

Prep Time: 5 minutes

Servings: 1

Day 2

Breakfast: Berry Spinach Smoothie

Ingredients:

- 1 cup fresh spinach

- 1/2 cup mixed berries (strawberries, blueberries, raspberries)

- 1/2 banana

- 1/2 cup unsweetened almond milk or water

- 1 tablespoon chia seeds (optional)

- Ice cubes

Preparation:

1. Combine all ingredients in a blender.

2. Blend until smooth and creamy.

3. Add more liquid if needed to reach desired consistency.

4. Pour into a glass and serve immediately.

Prep Time: 5 minutes

Servings: 1

Lunch: Quinoa Salad with Grilled Vegetables

Ingredients:

- 1/2 cup cooked quinoa

- 1 cup mixed grilled vegetables (bell peppers, zucchini, eggplant)

- 2 tablespoons crumbled feta cheese

- 1 tablespoon chopped fresh parsley

- 1 tablespoon balsamic vinaigrette

Preparation:

1. Cook quinoa according to package instructions and let it cool.

2. Grill mixed vegetables until tender and slightly charred.

3. In a bowl, combine cooked quinoa, grilled vegetables, crumbled feta cheese, chopped parsley, and balsamic vinaigrette.

4. Toss gently to mix well.

5. Serve chilled or at room temperature.

Prep Time: 15 minutes

Servings: 1

Dinner: Lemon Herb Chicken with Roasted Sweet Potatoes and Green Beans

Ingredients:

- 1 boneless, skinless chicken breast

- 1 tablespoon olive oil

- 1 tablespoon lemon juice

- 1 teaspoon chopped fresh rosemary

- 1 teaspoon chopped fresh thyme

- Salt and pepper to taste

- 1 medium sweet potato, peeled and cubed

- 1 cup green beans, trimmed

- 1/2 tablespoon balsamic glaze (optional)

Cooking Directions:

1. Preheat oven to 400°F (200°C).

2. In a small bowl, mix olive oil, lemon juice, chopped rosemary, chopped thyme, salt, and pepper.

3. Rub the chicken breast with the herb mixture.

4. Place sweet potato cubes and green beans on a baking sheet.

5. Drizzle with olive oil and season with salt and pepper.

6. Place the chicken breast on the baking sheet with vegetables.

7. Bake for 20-25 minutes or until chicken is cooked through and vegetables are tender.

8. Drizzle with balsamic glaze before serving if desired.

Prep Time: 15 minutes

Cook Time: 20-25 minutes

Servings: 1

Snack: Greek Yogurt with Almonds and Honey

Ingredients:

- 1/2 cup plain Greek yogurt

- 1 tablespoon sliced almonds

- 1 teaspoon honey

Preparation:

1. Place Greek yogurt in a bowl.

2. Top with sliced almonds and drizzle with honey.

3. Mix well before enjoying.

Prep Time: 2 minutes

Servings: 1

Day 3

Breakfast:Avocado Toast with Poached Egg

Ingredients:

- 1 slice whole grain bread, toasted

- 1/4 avocado, mashed

- 1 poached egg

- Salt and pepper to taste

Preparation:

1. Spread mashed avocado on toasted bread.

2. Top with a poached egg.

3. Season with salt and pepper to taste.

Prep Time: 10 minutes (including poaching egg)

Servings: 1

Lunch: Salmon Salad with Mixed Greens

Ingredients:

- 4 oz cooked salmon, flaked

- 2 cups mixed greens (spinach, kale, arugula)

- 1/4 cup cherry tomatoes, halved

- 1/4 cup sliced cucumber

- 1/4 avocado, sliced

- 1 tablespoon chopped fresh dill

- 1 tablespoon extra virgin olive oil

- 1 tablespoon lemon juice

- Salt and pepper to taste

Preparation:

1. In a bowl, combine mixed greens, cherry tomatoes, sliced cucumber, sliced avocado, and flaked salmon.

2. Drizzle with olive oil and lemon juice.

3. Season with salt, pepper, and chopped fresh dill.

4. Toss gently to coat.

5. Serve immediately.

Prep Time: 10 minutes

Servings: 1

Dinner: Vegetable Curry with Brown Rice

Ingredients:

- 1 tablespoon olive oil

- 1/2 onion, diced

- 2 cloves garlic, minced

- 1 tablespoon grated ginger

- 1 tablespoon curry powder

- 1 cup mixed vegetables (carrots, bell peppers, peas)

- 1 cup coconut milk

- Salt and pepper to taste

- 1 cup cooked brown rice

Cooking Directions:

1. Heat olive oil in a skillet over medium heat.

2. Add diced onion, minced garlic, and grated ginger. Cook until fragrant.

3. Stir in curry powder and cook for another minute.

4. Add mixed vegetables and cook until tender.

5. Pour in coconut milk and bring to a simmer.

6. Season with salt and pepper to taste.

7. Serve vegetable curry over cooked brown rice.

Prep Time: 15 minutes

Cook Time: 20 minutes

Servings: 2

Snack: Apple Slices with Almond Butter

Ingredients:

- 1 apple, sliced

- 2 tablespoons almond butter

Preparation:

1. Spread almond butter on apple slices.

2. Enjoy as a tasty and nutritious snack.

Prep Time: 5 minutes

Servings: 1

Day 4

Breakfast:Blueberry Chia Seed Smoothie

Ingredients:

- 1/2 cup blueberries

- 1 tablespoon chia seeds

- 1/2 banana

- 1/2 cup unsweetened almond milk or water

- 1 tablespoon honey or maple syrup (optional)

- Ice cubes

Preparation:

1. Combine all ingredients in a blender.

2. Blend until smooth and creamy.

3. Add more liquid if needed to achieve desired consistency.

4. Pour into a glass and serve immediately.

Prep Time: 5 minutes

Servings: 1

Lunch: Spinach and Strawberry Salad with Grilled Chicken

Ingredients:

- 2 cups baby spinach

- 1/2 cup sliced strawberries

- 1/4 cup sliced almonds

- 3 oz grilled chicken breast, sliced

- 1 tablespoon balsamic vinaigrette

Preparation:

1. In a large bowl, combine baby spinach, sliced strawberries, sliced almonds, and grilled chicken slices.

2. Drizzle with balsamic vinaigrette.

3. Toss gently to coat.

4. Serve immediately.

Prep Time: 10 minutes (if chicken is pre-cooked)

Servings: 1

Dinner: Lentil and Vegetable Soup

Ingredients:

- 1 tablespoon olive oil

- 1/2 onion, diced

- 2 carrots, diced

- 2 celery stalks, diced

- 2 cloves garlic, minced

- 1 cup dried green lentils, rinsed

- 4 cups vegetable broth

- 1 teaspoon ground cumin

- 1/2 teaspoon paprika

- Salt and pepper to taste

- Chopped fresh parsley for garnish

Cooking Directions:

1. Heat olive oil in a large pot over medium heat.

2. Add diced onion, carrots, and celery. Cook until softened.

3. Stir in minced garlic and cook for another minute.

4. Add rinsed lentils, vegetable broth, ground cumin, paprika, salt, and pepper.

5. Bring to a boil, then reduce heat and simmer for 25-30 minutes or until lentils are tender.

6. Adjust seasoning if needed.

7. Garnish with chopped fresh parsley before serving.

Prep Time: 10 minutes

Cook Time: 30 minutes

Servings: 4

Snack: Greek Yogurt with Berries

Ingredients:

- 1/2 cup plain Greek yogurt

- 1/4 cup mixed berries (strawberries, blueberries, raspberries)

Preparation:

1. Spoon Greek yogurt into a bowl.

2. Top with mixed berries.

3. Enjoy as a refreshing snack.

Prep Time: 2 minutes

Servings: 1

Day 5

Breakfast: Overnight Chia Seed Pudding

Ingredients:

- 2 tablespoons chia seeds

- 1/2 cup unsweetened almond milk or coconut milk

- 1/2 teaspoon vanilla extract

- 1 teaspoon honey or maple syrup (optional)

- Sliced fruits for topping (such as berries, banana)

- Chopped nuts for topping (such as almonds, walnuts)

Preparation:

1. In a bowl or jar, mix chia seeds, almond milk, vanilla extract, and honey (if using).

2. Stir well to combine.

3. Cover and refrigerate overnight, or for at least 4 hours, until the mixture thickens and forms a pudding-like consistency.

4. Before serving, top with sliced fruits and chopped nuts.

Prep Time: 5 minutes (+ chilling time)

Servings: 1

Lunch: Quinoa and Black Bean Salad

Ingredients:

- 1/2 cup cooked quinoa

- 1/2 cup canned black beans, drained and rinsed

- 1/4 cup diced red bell pepper

- 1/4 cup diced cucumber

- 2 tablespoons chopped fresh cilantro

- 1 tablespoon lime juice

- 1 tablespoon extra virgin olive oil

- Salt and pepper to taste

- Avocado slices for serving (optional)

Preparation:

1. In a bowl, combine cooked quinoa, black beans, diced red bell pepper, diced cucumber, and chopped cilantro.

2. Drizzle with lime juice and olive oil.

3. Season with salt and pepper.

4. Toss gently to combine.

5. Serve with avocado slices on top if desired.

Prep Time: 10 minutes

Servings: 1

Dinner: Baked Chicken Thighs with Roasted Vegetables

Ingredients:

- 2 bone-in, skin-on chicken thighs

- 1 tablespoon olive oil

- 1 teaspoon paprika

- 1/2 teaspoon garlic powder

- 1/2 teaspoon dried thyme

- Salt and pepper to taste

- 1 cup mixed vegetables (such as carrots, broccoli, cauliflower)

- 1/2 tablespoon balsamic vinegar

Cooking Directions:

1. Preheat oven to 400°F (200°C).

2. In a small bowl, mix olive oil, paprika, garlic powder, dried thyme, salt, and pepper.

3. Rub the chicken thighs with the spice mixture.

4. Place chicken thighs on a baking sheet lined with parchment paper.

5. Arrange mixed vegetables around the chicken thighs.

6. Drizzle vegetables with balsamic vinegar.

7. Bake for 25-30 minutes or until chicken is cooked through and vegetables are tender.

Prep Time: 10 minutes

Cook Time: 25-30 minutes

Servings: 2

Snack: Celery Sticks with Almond Butter

Ingredients:

- 2 celery stalks, cut into sticks

- 2 tablespoons almond butter

Preparation:

1. Spread almond butter on celery sticks.

2. Enjoy as a crunchy and satisfying snack.

Prep Time: 5 minutes

Servings: 1

Day 6

Breakfast:Banana Almond Butter Toast

Ingredients:

- 1 slice whole grain bread, toasted

- 1 tablespoon almond butter

- 1/2 banana, sliced

- 1 teaspoon honey (optional)

Preparation:

1. Spread almond butter evenly on the toasted whole grain bread.

2. Top with sliced banana.

3. Drizzle with honey if desired.

Prep Time: 5 minutes

Servings: 1

Lunch: Grilled Vegetable Wrap

Ingredients:

- 1 whole grain wrap

- 1/2 cup mixed grilled vegetables (zucchini, bell peppers, eggplant)

- 2 tablespoons hummus

- Handful of mixed greens

- Salt and pepper to taste

Preparation:

1. Spread hummus evenly on the whole grain wrap.

2. Layer with mixed grilled vegetables and mixed greens.

3. Season with salt and pepper to taste.

4. Roll up tightly and slice in half.

Prep Time: 10 minutes

Servings: 1

Dinner: Herb-Roasted Pork Tenderloin with Quinoa and Steamed Green Beans

Ingredients:

- 1 pork tenderloin (about 8 oz)zoregano

- Salt and pepper to taste

- 1 cup cooked quinoa

- 1 cup steamed green beans

Cooking Directions:

1. Preheat oven to 400°F (200°C).

2. Rub the pork tenderloin with olive oil, dried thyme, dried rosemary, dried oregano, salt, and pepper.

3. Place the pork tenderloin on a baking sheet lined with parchment paper.

4. Roast in the oven for 20-25 minutes or until the internal temperature reaches 145°F (63°C).

5. Remove from the oven and let it rest for 5 minutes before slicing.

6. Serve the sliced pork tenderloin with cooked quinoa and steamed green beans.

Prep Time: 10 minutes

Cook Time: 20-25 minutes

Servings: 2

Snack: Mixed Nuts and Dried Fruits

Ingredients:

- 1/4 cup mixed nuts (such as almonds, walnuts, cashews)

- 1/4 cup dried fruits (such as apricots, raisins, cranberries)

Preparation:

1. Mix the mixed nuts and dried fruits in a bowl.

2. Enjoy as a nutritious and satisfying snack.

Prep Time: 2 minutes

Servings:

Day 7

Breakfast: Greek Yogurt Parfait

Ingredients:

- 1/2 cup plain Greek yogurt

- 1/4 cup granola (low-sodium, if available)

- 1/4 cup mixed berries (strawberries, blueberries, raspberries)

- 1 tablespoon honey (optional)

Preparation:

1. In a glass or bowl, layer Greek yogurt, granola, and mixed berries.

2. Drizzle with honey if desired.

Prep Time: 5 minutes

Servings: 1

Lunch: Quinoa and Chickpea Buddha Bowl

Ingredients:

- 1/2 cup cooked quinoa

- 1/2 cup cooked chickpeas

- 1/2 cup roasted sweet potato cubes

- 1/2 cup steamed broccoli florets

- 1/4 avocado, sliced

- 1 tablespoon tahini dressing

- Sesame seeds for garnish (optional)

Preparation:

1. In a bowl, arrange cooked quinoa, cooked chickpeas, roasted sweet potato cubes, and steamed broccoli florets.

2. Top with sliced avocado.

3. Drizzle with tahini dressing.

4. Garnish with sesame seeds if desired.

Prep Time: 15 minutes

Servings: 1

Dinner: **Mediterranean Stuffed Bell Peppers**

Ingredients:

- 2 bell peppers, halved and seeds removed

- 1/2 cup cooked quinoa

- 1/2 cup canned chickpeas, drained and rinsed

- 1/4 cup diced tomatoes

- 1/4 cup chopped cucumber

- 2 tablespoons crumbled feta cheese

- 1 tablespoon chopped fresh parsley

- 1 tablespoon lemon juice

- Salt and pepper to taste

- Olive oil for drizzling

Cooking Directions:

1. Preheat oven to 375°F (190°C).

2. In a bowl, mix cooked quinoa, chickpeas, diced tomatoes, chopped cucumber, crumbled feta cheese, chopped parsley, lemon juice, salt, and pepper.

3. Stuff bell pepper halves with the quinoa mixture.

4. Drizzle with olive oil.

5. Place stuffed peppers on a baking sheet and bake for 25-30 minutes until peppers are tender.

Prep Time: 15 minutes

Cook Time: 25-30 minutes

Servings: 2

Snack: Sliced Apple with Peanut Butter

Ingredients:

- 1 apple, sliced

- 2 tablespoons peanut butter

Preparation:

1. Spread peanut butter on apple slices.

2. Enjoy as a delicious and satisfying snack.

Prep Time: 2 minutes

Servings: 1

Day 8

Breakfast:Spinach and Mushroom Omelette

Ingredients:

- 2 eggs

- 1/4 cup chopped spinach

- 1/4 cup sliced mushrooms

- 1 tablespoon grated Parmesan cheese

- Salt and pepper to taste

- 1 teaspoon olive oil

Preparation:

1. In a bowl, whisk eggs with salt, pepper, and grated Parmesan cheese.

2. Heat olive oil in a non-stick skillet over medium heat.

3. Add sliced mushrooms and sauté until softened.

4. Add chopped spinach to the skillet and cook until wilted.

5. Pour the egg mixture into the skillet with mushrooms and spinach.

6. Cook until the edges are set, then gently lift the edges and tilt the skillet to let the uncooked egg flow to the bottom.

7. Once the omelette is cooked through, fold it in half and slide onto a plate.

8. Serve hot.

Prep Time: 10 minutes

Cook Time: 5 minutes

Servings: 1

Lunch: Lentil Salad with Roasted Vegetables

Ingredients:

- 1/2 cup cooked lentils

- 1 cup mixed roasted vegetables (such as carrots, bell peppers, onions)

- 2 tablespoons crumbled goat cheese

- 1 tablespoon balsamic vinaigrette

- Fresh basil leaves for garnish (optional)

Preparation:

1. In a bowl, combine cooked lentils and mixed roasted vegetables.

2. Add crumbled goat cheese and balsamic vinaigrette.

3. Toss gently to combine.

4. Garnish with fresh basil leaves if desired.

5. Serve at room temperature or chilled.

Prep Time: 15 minutes

Servings: 1

Dinner: Baked Cod with Lemon Herb Sauce and Steamed Asparagus

Ingredients:

- 2 cod fillets

- 1 tablespoon olive oil

- 1 teaspoon chopped fresh parsley

- 1 teaspoon chopped fresh dill

- 1 clove garlic, minced

- Zest and juice of 1 lemon

- Salt and pepper to taste

- 1 bunch asparagus, trimmed

- Lemon wedges for serving

Cooking Directions:

1. Preheat oven to 375°F (190°C).

2. Place cod fillets on a baking sheet lined with parchment paper.

3. In a small bowl, mix olive oil, chopped parsley, chopped dill, minced garlic, lemon zest, lemon juice, salt, and pepper.

4. Brush the herb mixture over the cod fillets.

5. Bake for 15-20 minutes or until the fish flakes easily with a fork.

6. While the fish is baking, steam the asparagus until tender.

7. Serve the baked cod with steamed asparagus and lemon wedges.

Prep Time: 10 minutes

Cook Time: 15-20 minutes

Servings: 2

Snack: Cucumber Slices with Hummus

Ingredients:

- 1/2 cucumber, sliced

- 2 tablespoons hummus

Preparation:

1. Dip cucumber slices into hummus.

2. Enjoy as a refreshing and crunchy snack.

Prep Time: 5 minutes

Servings: 1

Day 9

Breakfast: Berry Protein Smoothie

Ingredients:

- 1/2 cup mixed berries (strawberries, blueberries, raspberries)

- 1/2 banana

- 1/2 cup plain Greek yogurt

- 1/2 cup unsweetened almond milk or water

- 1 scoop protein powder (optional)

- Ice cubes

Preparation:

1. Combine all ingredients in a blender.

2. Blend until smooth and creamy.

3. Add more liquid if needed to reach desired consistency.

4. Pour into a glass and enjoy.

Prep Time: 5 minutes

Servings: 1

Lunch: Mediterranean Chickpea Salad

Ingredients:

- 1 cup canned chickpeas, drained and rinsed

- 1/2 cup diced cucumber

- 1/2 cup cherry tomatoes, halved

- 1/4 cup diced red onion

- 2 tablespoons chopped fresh parsley

- 2 tablespoons crumbled feta cheese

- 1 tablespoon extra virgin olive oil

- 1 tablespoon lemon juice

- Salt and pepper to taste

Preparation:

1. In a large bowl, combine chickpeas, cucumber, cherry tomatoes, red onion, parsley, and feta cheese.

2. Drizzle with olive oil and lemon juice.

3. Season with salt and pepper.

4. Toss gently to combine.

5. Serve chilled or at room temperature.

Prep Time: 10 minutes

Servings: 2

Dinner: Turkey and Vegetable Stir-Fry

Ingredients:

- 1 tablespoon olive oil

- 8 oz turkey breast, thinly sliced

- 2 cups mixed vegetables (bell peppers, broccoli, snap peas, carrots)

- 2 tablespoons low-sodium soy sauce

- 1 tablespoon hoisin sauce

- 1 teaspoon grated ginger

- 2 cloves garlic, minced

- Cooked brown rice for serving

Cooking Directions:

1. Heat olive oil in a large skillet or wok over medium-high heat.

2. Add sliced turkey breast and cook until browned and cooked through.

3. Remove turkey from the skillet and set aside.

4. In the same skillet, add mixed vegetables and stir-fry until tender-crisp.

5. Return cooked turkey to the skillet.

6. In a small bowl, mix soy sauce, hoisin sauce, grated ginger, and minced garlic.

7. Pour the sauce over the turkey and vegetables in the skillet.

8. Cook for an additional 2-3 minutes, stirring constantly.

9. Serve hot over cooked brown rice.

Prep Time: 15 minutes

Cook Time: 15 minutes

Servings: 2

Snack: Greek Yogurt with Honey and Almonds

Ingredients:

- 1/2 cup plain Greek yogurt

- 1 tablespoon honey

- 1 tablespoon sliced almonds

Preparation:

1. Spoon Greek yogurt into a bowl.

2. Drizzle with honey and sprinkle sliced almonds on top.

3. Enjoy as a creamy and satisfying snack.

Prep Time: 2 minutes

Servings: 1

Day 10

Breakfast: Avocado Breakfast Toast

Ingredients:

- 1 slice whole grain bread, toasted

- 1/2 ripe avocado, mashed

- 1 poached egg

- Pinch of red pepper flakes (optional)

- Salt and pepper to taste

Preparation:

1. Spread mashed avocado evenly on the toasted whole grain bread.

2. Top with a poached egg.

3. Sprinkle with red pepper flakes if desired.

4. Season with salt and pepper.

5. Serve hot.

Prep Time: 10 minutes

Servings: 1

Lunch: Quinoa and Black Bean Stuffed Bell Peppers

Ingredients:

- 2 bell peppers, halved and seeds removed

- 1 cup cooked quinoa

- 1 cup canned black beans, drained and rinsed

- 1/2 cup diced tomatoess

- 1/4 cup chopped red onion

- 1/4 cup shredded cheddar cheese

- 1 teaspoon chili powder

- 1/2 teaspoon ground cumin

- Salt and pepper to taste

Cooking Directions:

1. Preheat oven to 375°F (190°C).

2. In a large bowl, mix cooked quinoa, black beans, diced tomatoes, chopped red onion, shredded cheddar cheese, chili powder, ground cumin, salt, and pepper.

3. Stuff bell pepper halves with the quinoa and black bean mixture.

4. Place stuffed peppers on a baking sheet lined with parchment paper.

5. Bake for 25-30 minutes or until peppers are tender and filling is heated through.

Prep Time: 15 minutes

Cook Time: 25-30 minutes

Servings: 2

Dinner: Salmon with Roasted Brussels Sprouts and Sweet Potatoes

Ingredients:

- 2 salmon fillets

- 1 tablespoon olive oil

- 1 teaspoon lemon zest

- 1 tablespoon lemon juice

- 1 teaspoon chopped fresh dill

- Salt and pepper to taste

- 1 cup Brussels sprouts, trimmed and halved

- 1 medium sweet potato, peeled and diced

- 1 tablespoon balsamic glaze (optional)

Cooking Directions:

1. Preheat oven to 400°F (200°C).

2. In a small bowl, mix olive oil, lemon zest, lemon juice, chopped dill, salt, and pepper.

3. Place salmon fillets on a baking sheet lined with parchment paper.

4. Brush the lemon-dill mixture over the salmon.

5. Arrange Brussels sprouts and diced sweet potatoes around the salmon on the baking sheet.

6. Drizzle vegetables with olive oil and season with salt and pepper.

7. Bake for 15-20 minutes or until salmon is cooked through and vegetables are tender.

8. Drizzle with balsamic glaze before serving if desired.

Prep Time: 15 minutes

Cook Time: 15-20 minutes

Servings: 2

Snack: Carrot and Celery Sticks with Hummus

Ingredients:

- 1 carrot, cut into sticks

- 1 celery stalk, cut into sticks

- 2 tablespoons hummus

Preparation:

1. Dip carrot and celery sticks into hummus.

2. Enjoy as a crunchy and nutritious snack.

Prep Time: 5 minutes

Servings: 1

Day 11

Breakfast: Spinach and Feta Breakfast Wrap

Ingredients:

- 1 whole grain wrap

- 1/4 cup cooked quinoa

- Handful of fresh spinach leaves

- 2 tablespoons crumbled feta cheese

- 1 tablespoon chopped sun-dried tomatoes (optional)

- Salt and pepper to taste

- Olive oil cooking spray

Preparation:

1. Heat a non-stick skillet over medium heat and lightly coat with olive oil cooking spray.

2. Place the wrap on the skillet and warm for about 1 minute on each side.

3. In the center of the wrap, layer cooked quinoa, fresh spinach leaves, crumbled feta cheese, and chopped sun-dried tomatoes (if using).

4. Season with salt and pepper to taste.

5. Fold in the sides of the wrap and roll it up tightly.

6. Return the wrap to the skillet and cook for an additional 2 minutes on each side until lightly golden and crispy.

7. Serve warm.

Prep Time: 10 minutes

Cook Time: 5 minutes

Servings: 1

Lunch: Mediterranean Tuna Salad

Ingredients:

- 1 can (5 oz) tuna, drained

- 1/4 cup diced cucumber

- 1/4 cup diced tomatoes

- 2 tablespoons sliced Kalamata olives

- 1 tablespoon chopped red onion

- 1 tablespoon chopped fresh parsley

- 1 tablespoon extra virgin olive oil

- 1 tablespoon lemon juice

- Salt and pepper to taste

- Whole grain pita bread or lettuce leaves for serving

Preparation:

1. In a bowl, combine drained tuna, diced cucumber, diced tomatoes, sliced Kalamata olives, chopped red onion, and chopped fresh parsley.

2. Drizzle with olive oil and lemon juice.

3. Season with salt and pepper.

4. Toss gently to combine.

5. Serve the Mediterranean tuna salad with whole grain pita bread or wrapped in lettuce leaves.

Prep Time: 10 minutes

Servings: 1

Dinner: Vegetable and Lentil Curry

Ingredients:

- 1 tablespoon olive oil

- 1/2 onion, diced

- 2 cloves garlic, minced

- 1 tablespoon grated ginger

- 1 tablespoon curry powder

- 1 cup cooked lentils

- 1 can (14 oz) diced tomatoes

- 2 cups mixed vegetables (such as cauliflower, bell peppers, carrots)

- 1 cup coconut milk

- Salt and pepper to taste

- Cooked brown rice for serving

Cooking Directions:

1. Heat olive oil in a large skillet over medium heat.

2. Add diced onion and cook until softened.

3. Stir in minced garlic, grated ginger, and curry powder. Cook for another minute.

4. Add cooked lentils, diced tomatoes, mixed vegetables, and coconut milk.

5. Bring to a simmer and cook for 15-20 minutes, stirring occasionally, until vegetables are tender.

6. Season with salt and pepper to taste.

7. Serve vegetable and lentil curry over cooked brown rice.

Prep Time: 15 minutes

Cook Time: 20 minutes

Servings: 2

Snack: Sliced Pear with Almond Butter

Ingredients:

- 1 pear, sliced

- 2 tablespoons almond butter

Preparation:

1. Spread almond butter on pear slices.

2. Enjoy as a delicious and nutritious snack.

Prep Time: 2 minutes

Servings: 1

Day 12

Breakfast: Veggie and Cheese Omelette

Ingredients:

- 2 eggs

- 1/4 cup diced bell peppers (any color)

- 1/4 cup diced tomatoes

- 2 tablespoons diced onions

- 2 tablespoons shredded cheese (cheddar, mozzarella, or your choice)

- Salt and pepper to taste

- 1 teaspoon olive oil

Preparation:

1. In a bowl, beat the eggs until well combined. Season with salt and pepper.

2. Heat olive oil in a non-stick skillet over medium heat.

3. Add diced bell peppers, tomatoes, and onions to the skillet. Cook until softened.

4. Pour the beaten eggs over the cooked vegetables in the skillet.

5. Sprinkle shredded cheese on top.

6. Cook until the edges are set and the bottom is golden brown.

7. Flip the omelette and cook for another minute until cooked through.

8. Fold the omelette in half and transfer to a plate.

9. Serve hot.

Prep Time: 10 minutes

Cook Time: 5 minutes

Servings: 1

Lunch: Quinoa Salad with Lemon Herb Dressing

Ingredients:

- 1 cup cooked quinoa

- 1/2 cup diced cucumber

- 1/2 cup halved cherry tomatoes

- 1/4 cup chopped fresh parsley

- 2 tablespoons chopped fresh mint

- 1 tablespoon extra virgin olive oil

- 1 tablespoon lemon juice

- Salt and pepper to taste

- Crumbled feta cheese for garnish (optional)

Preparation:

1. In a large bowl, combine cooked quinoa, diced cucumber, halved cherry tomatoes, chopped fresh parsley, and chopped fresh mint.

2. In a small bowl, whisk together olive oil, lemon juice, salt, and pepper to make the dressing.

3. Drizzle the dressing over the quinoa salad and toss gently to combine.

4. Garnish with crumbled feta cheese if desired.

5. Serve chilled or at room temperature.

Prep Time: 15 minutes

Servings: 2

Dinner: Grilled Chicken with Roasted Vegetables

Ingredients:

- 2 boneless, skinless chicken breasts

- 1 tablespoon olive oil

- 1 teaspoon dried Italian herbs (basil, oregano, thyme)

- Salt and pepper to taste

- 2 cups mixed vegetables (such as bell peppers, zucchini, red onion, mushrooms)

- 1 tablespoon balsamic vinegar

- Fresh parsley for garnish

Cooking Directions:

1. Preheat grill to medium-high heat.

2. Brush chicken breasts with olive oil and season with dried Italian herbs, salt, and pepper.

3. Grill chicken for 6-8 minutes per side or until cooked through.

4. In the meantime, toss mixed vegetables with olive oil, balsamic vinegar, salt, and pepper.

5. Spread vegetables on a baking sheet lined with parchment paper.

6. Roast in the oven at 400°F (200°C) for 15-20 minutes or until tender.

7. Serve grilled chicken with roasted vegetables, garnished with fresh parsley.

Prep Time: 15 minutes

Cook Time: 25-30 minutes

Servings: 2

Snack: Greek Yogurt with Granola

Ingredients:

- 1/2 cup plain Greek yogurt

- 1/4 cup granola (low-sugar, if available)

- Mixed berries for topping (optional)

Preparation:

1. Spoon Greek yogurt into a bowl.

2. Sprinkle granola on top.

3. Add mixed berries for extra flavor and nutrients if desired.

4. Enjoy as a satisfying snack.

Prep Time: 2 minutes

Servings: 1

Day 13

Breakfast: Berry Almond Smoothie Bowl

Ingredients:

- 1/2 cup frozen mixed berries (strawberries, blueberries, raspberries)

- 1/2 banana

- 1/2 cup unsweetened almond milk

- 1 tablespoon almond butter

- 1 tablespoon chia seeds

- Toppings: sliced almonds, fresh berries, granola (optional)

Preparation:

1. In a blender, combine frozen mixed berries, banana, almond milk, almond butter, and chia seeds.

2. Blend until smooth and creamy.

3. Pour the smoothie into a bowl.

4. Top with sliced almonds, fresh berries, and granola if desired.

5. Enjoy with a spoon!

Prep Time: 5 minutes

Servings: 1

Lunch: Chickpea Salad Sandwich

Ingredients:

- 1/2 cup canned chickpeas, drained and rinsed

- 2 tablespoons diced celery

- 2 tablespoons diced red onion

- 1 tablespoon chopped fresh parsley

- 1 tablespoon lemon juice

- 1 tablespoon plain Greek yogurt

- Salt and pepper to taste

- 2 slices whole grain bread

- Lettuce leaves and sliced tomatoes for serving

Preparation:

1. In a bowl, mash the chickpeas with a fork.

2. Add diced celery, diced red onion, chopped fresh parsley, lemon juice, Greek yogurt, salt, and pepper to the mashed chickpeas. Mix well.

3. Toast the whole grain bread slices if desired.

4. Place lettuce leaves and sliced tomatoes on one slice of bread.

5. Spoon the chickpea salad mixture over the lettuce and tomatoes.

6. Top with the other slice of bread to make a sandwich.

7. Cut the sandwich in half if desired.

8. Serve and enjoy!

Prep Time: 10 minutes

Servings: 1

Dinner: Vegetable and Tofu Stir-Fry with Brown Rice

Ingredients:

- 1 tablespoon sesame oil

- 8 oz firm tofu, cubed

- 2 cups mixed vegetables (such as bell peppers, broccoli, snap peas, carrots)

- 2 tablespoons low-sodium soy sauce

- 1 tablespoon hoisin sauce

- 1 teaspoon grated ginger

- 2 cloves garlic, minced

- Cooked brown rice for serving

Cooking Directions:

1. Heat sesame oil in a large skillet or wok over medium-high heat.

2. Add cubed tofu to the skillet and cook until golden brown on all sides.

3. Remove tofu from the skillet and set aside.

4. In the same skillet, add mixed vegetables and stir-fry until tender-crisp.

5. Return cooked tofu to the skillet.

6. In a small bowl, mix soy sauce, hoisin sauce, grated ginger, and minced garlic.

7. Pour the sauce over the tofu and vegetables in the skillet.

8. Cook for an additional 2-3 minutes, stirring constantly.

9. Serve hot over cooked brown rice.

Prep Time: 15 minutes

Cook Time: 15 minutes

Servings: 2

Snack: Celery Sticks with Cashew Cream Cheese

Ingredients:

- 2 celery stalks, cut into sticks

- 2 tablespoons cashew cream cheese (or any non-dairy cream cheese)

Preparation:

1. Spread cashew cream cheese on celery sticks.

2. Enjoy as a crunchy and satisfying snack.

Prep Time: 5 minutes

Servings: 1

Day 14

Breakfast: Greek Yogurt Parfait with Nuts and Berries

Ingredients:

- 1/2 cup plain Greek yogurt

- 1/4 cup granola (low-sugar, if available)

- 1/4 cup mixed berries (such as strawberries, blueberries, raspberries)

- 1 tablespoon chopped nuts (such as almonds, walnuts, or pecans)

- Drizzle of honey or maple syrup (optional)

Preparation:

1. In a glass or bowl, layer Greek yogurt, granola, mixed berries, and chopped nuts.

2. Drizzle with honey or maple syrup if desired.

3. Serve and enjoy!

Prep Time: 5 minutes

Servings: 1

Lunch: Lentil and Vegetable Soup

Ingredients:

- 1 tablespoon olive oil

- 1/2 onion, diced

- 2 cloves garlic, minced

- 2 carrots, diced

- 2 celery stalks, diced

- 1 cup dried green or brown lentils, rinsed and drained

- 4 cups vegetable broth

- 1 can (14 oz) diced tomatoes

- 1 teaspoon dried thyme

- Salt and pepper to taste

- Fresh parsley for garnish

Cooking Directions:

1. Heat olive oil in a large pot over medium heat.

2. Add diced onion and minced garlic to the pot. Cook until softened.

3. Stir in diced carrots and celery. Cook for another 5 minutes.

4. Add dried lentils, vegetable broth, diced tomatoes, and dried thyme to the pot.

5. Season with salt and pepper to taste.

6. Bring the soup to a boil, then reduce heat to low and simmer for 25-30 minutes or until lentils are tender.

7. Serve hot, garnished with fresh parsley.

Prep Time: 10 minutes

Cook Time: 30 minutes

Servings: 4

Dinner: Baked Salmon with Lemon-Dill Sauce and Steamed Vegetables

Ingredients:

- 2 salmon fillets

- 1 tablespoon olive oil

- 1 teaspoon dried dill

- Zest and juice of 1 lemon

- Salt and pepper to taste

- Mixed vegetables for steaming (such as broccoli, cauliflower, carrots)

Cooking Directions:

1. Preheat oven to 375°F (190°C).

2. Place salmon fillets on a baking sheet lined with parchment paper.

3. In a small bowl, mix olive oil, dried dill, lemon zest, lemon juice, salt, and pepper.

4. Brush the lemon-dill mixture over the salmon.

5. Bake for 15-20 minutes or until the salmon is cooked through and flakes easily with a fork.

6. While the salmon is baking, steam mixed vegetables until tender.

7. Serve baked salmon with steamed vegetables.

Prep Time: 10 minutes

Cook Time: 15-20 minutes

Servings: 2

Snack: Rice Cakes with Avocado Mash

Ingredients:

- 2 rice cakes

- 1/2 avocado, mashed

- Pinch of red pepper flakes (optional)

- Salt and pepper to taste

Preparation:

1. Spread mashed avocado evenly on the rice cakes.

2. Sprinkle with red pepper flakes, salt, and pepper.

3. Enjoy as a satisfying and crunchy snack.

Prep Time: 5 minutes

Servings: 1

Day 15

Breakfast: Banana Nut Oatmeal

Ingredients:

- 1/2 cup rolled oats

- 1 cup water or milk of your choice

- 1 ripe banana, mashed

- 1 tablespoon chopped nuts (such as almonds, walnuts, or pecans)

- Pinch of cinnamon

- Drizzle of honey or maple syrup (optional)

Preparation:

1. In a small saucepan, bring water or milk to a boil.

2. Stir in rolled oats and reduce heat to low. Cook for 5-7 minutes, stirring occasionally, until oats are creamy.

3. Stir in mashed banana, chopped nuts, and a pinch of cinnamon.

4. Cook for another 1-2 minutes until heated through.

5. If desired, drizzle with honey or maple syrup for sweetness.

6. Serve hot.

Prep Time: 2 minutes

Cook Time: 7 minutes

Servings: 1

Lunch: Quinoa and Black Bean Salad

Ingredients:

- 1 cup cooked quinoa

- 1 cup canned black beans, drained and rinsed

- 1/2 cup diced bell peppers (any color)

- 1/4 cup diced red onion

- 1/4 cup chopped fresh cilantro

- 2 tablespoons lime juice

- 1 tablespoon extra virgin olive oil

- Salt and pepper to taste

- Avocado slices for serving (optional)

Preparation:

1. In a large bowl, combine cooked quinoa, black beans, diced bell peppers, diced red onion, and chopped fresh cilantro.

2. In a small bowl, whisk together lime juice, olive oil, salt, and pepper to make the dressing.

3. Pour the dressing over the quinoa and black bean salad. Toss gently to combine.

4. Serve the salad at room temperature or chilled, garnished with avocado slices if desired.

Prep Time: 10 minutes

Servings: 2

Dinner: Lemon Herb Chicken with Roasted Vegetables

Ingredients:

- 2 boneless, skinless chicken breasts

- 2 tablespoons olive oil

- Zest and juice of 1 lemon

- 1 teaspoon dried thyme

- 1 teaspoon dried rosemary

- Salt and pepper to taste

- 2 cups mixed vegetables (such as carrots, Brussels sprouts, red potatoes)

- Fresh parsley for garnish

Cooking Directions:

1. Preheat oven to 400°F (200°C).

2. In a small bowl, mix olive oil, lemon zest, lemon juice, dried thyme, dried rosemary, salt, and pepper.

3. Place chicken breasts in a baking dish and brush with the lemon herb mixture.

4. Arrange mixed vegetables around the chicken in the baking dish.

5. Drizzle remaining lemon herb mixture over the vegetables.

6. Roast in the oven for 25-30 minutes or until chicken is cooked through and vegetables are tender.

7. Garnish with fresh parsley before serving.

Prep Time: 10 minutes

Cook Time: 25-30 minutes

Servings: 2

Snack: Apple Slices with Almond Butter

Ingredients:

- 1 apple, sliced

- 2 tablespoons almond butter

Preparation:

1. Spread almond butter on apple slices.

2. Enjoy as a delicious and nutritious snack.

Prep Time: 2 minutes

Servings: 1

Day 16

Breakfast: Veggie Breakfast Burrito

Ingredients:

- 2 large eggs

- 1/4 cup diced bell peppers (any color)

- 1/4 cup diced onions

- 1/4 cup diced tomatoes

- 1 tablespoon chopped fresh cilantro

- Salt and pepper to taste

- 1 whole grain tortilla

- 2 tablespoons shredded cheese (cheddar, mozzarella, or your choice)

- Salsa or hot sauce for serving (optional)

Preparation:

1. In a bowl, beat the eggs until well combined. Season with salt and pepper.

2. Heat a non-stick skillet over medium heat.

3. Add diced bell peppers and onions to the skillet. Cook until softened.

4. Stir in diced tomatoes and chopped fresh cilantro. Cook for another minute.

5. Pour the beaten eggs over the cooked vegetables in the skillet.

6. Cook, stirring occasionally, until the eggs are scrambled and cooked through.

7. Warm the whole grain tortilla in the skillet or microwave.

8. Spoon the scrambled eggs onto the tortilla.

9. Sprinkle shredded cheese on top.

10. Roll up the tortilla to make a burrito.

11. Serve with salsa or hot sauce if desired.

Prep Time: 10 minutes

Cook Time: 5 minutes

Servings: 1

Lunch: Spinach and Strawberry Salad with Balsamic Vinaigrette

Ingredients:

- 2 cups baby spinach leaves

- 1/2 cup sliced strawberries

- 2 tablespoons sliced almonds

- 2 tablespoons crumbled feta cheese

- 1 tablespoon balsamic vinegar

- 1 tablespoon extra virgin olive oil

- 1/2 teaspoon honey

- Salt and pepper to taste

Preparation:

1. In a large bowl, combine baby spinach leaves, sliced strawberries, sliced almonds, and crumbled feta cheese.

2. In a small bowl, whisk together balsamic vinegar, olive oil, honey, salt, and pepper to make the vinaigrette.

3. Drizzle the vinaigrette over the salad and toss gently to coat.

4. Serve immediately.

Prep Time: 10 minutes

Servings: 1

Dinner: Turkey and Vegetable Skewers with Quinoa

Ingredients:

- 8 oz turkey breast, cut into cubes

- 1 zucchini, cut into chunks

- 1 bell pepper, cut into chunks

- 1 onion, cut into chunks

- 1 tablespoon olive oil

- 1 teaspoon dried oregano

- 1 teaspoon paprika

- Salt and pepper to taste

- Cooked quinoa for serving

Cooking Directions:

1. Preheat grill or grill pan over medium-high heat.

2. Thread turkey cubes, zucchini chunks, bell pepper chunks, and onion chunks onto skewers.

3. In a small bowl, mix olive oil, dried oregano, paprika, salt, and pepper.

4. Brush the turkey and vegetable skewers with the olive oil mixture.

5. Grill skewers for 8-10 minutes, turning occasionally,

until turkey is cooked through and vegetables are tender.

6. Serve hot with cooked quinoa.

Prep Time: 15 minutes

Cook Time: 8-10 minutes

Servings: 2

Snack: **Cottage Cheese with Pineapple**

Ingredients:

- 1/2 cup low-fat cottage cheese

- 1/2 cup diced pineapple (fresh or canned in juice)

Preparation:

1. Spoon cottage cheese into a bowl.

2. Top with diced pineapple.

3. Enjoy as a protein-rich snack.

Prep Time: 2 minutes

Servings: 1

Day 17

Breakfast: **Blueberry Almond Smoothie**

Ingredients:

- 1/2 cup frozen blueberries

- 1/2 banana

- 1 tablespoon almond butter

- 1/2 cup unsweetened almond milk

- 1 tablespoon chia seeds

- Handful of spinach leaves (optional)

- Ice cubes (optional)

Preparation:

1. In a blender, combine frozen blueberries, banana, almond butter, almond milk, chia seeds, spinach leaves (if using), and ice cubes (if desired).

2. Blend until smooth and creamy.

3. Pour into a glass and serve immediately.

Prep Time: 5 minutes

Servings: 1

Lunch: Caprese Salad with Balsamic Glaze

Ingredients:

- 1 large ripe tomato, sliced

- 4-6 fresh basil leaves

- 2 oz fresh mozzarella cheese, sliced

- 1 tablespoon extra virgin olive oil

- 1 tablespoon balsamic glaze

- Salt and pepper to taste

Preparation:

1. Arrange tomato slices, fresh basil leaves, and mozzarella cheese slices on a plate.

2. Drizzle with extra virgin olive oil and balsamic glaze.

3. Season with salt and pepper to taste.

4. Serve immediately as a refreshing salad.

Prep Time: 5 minutes

Servings: 1

Dinner: Lentil Shepherd's Pie

Ingredients:

- 2 cups cooked lentils

- 1 tablespoon olive oil

- 1 onion, diced

- 2 carrots, diced

- 2 celery stalks, diced

- 2 cloves garlic, minced

- 1 teaspoon dried thyme

- 1 teaspoon dried rosemary

- Salt and pepper to taste

- 2 cups mashed potatoes (made from boiled potatoes)

- Fresh parsley for garnish

Cooking Directions:

1. Preheat oven to 375°F (190°C).

2. Heat olive oil in a large skillet over medium heat.

3. Add diced onion, carrots, and celery to the skillet. Cook until softened.

4. Stir in minced garlic, dried thyme, and dried rosemary. Cook for another minute.

5. Add cooked lentils to the skillet. Season with salt and pepper to taste. Cook until heated through.

6. Transfer the lentil mixture to a baking dish.

7. Spread mashed potatoes evenly over the lentil mixture.

8. Bake in the preheated oven for 25-30 minutes or until the top is golden brown.

9. Garnish with fresh parsley before serving.

Prep Time: 15 minutes

Cook Time: 25-30 minutes

Servings: 4

Snack: Whole Grain Crackers with Hummus

Ingredients:

- Whole grain crackers

- Hummus (store-bought or homemade)

Preparation:

1. Spread hummus on whole grain crackers.

2. Enjoy as a crunchy and satisfying snack.

Prep Time: 2 minutes

Servings: 1

Day 18

Breakfast: Avocado Toast with Poached Egg

Ingredients:

- 1 slice whole grain bread

- 1/2 avocado, mashed

- 1 egg

- Salt and pepper to taste

- Red pepper flakes for garnish (optional)

- Fresh herbs for garnish (optional)

Preparation:

1. Toast the whole grain bread until golden brown.

2. Spread mashed avocado evenly on the toast.

3. In a pot, bring water to a gentle simmer.

4. Crack the egg into a small bowl.

5. Create a whirlpool in the simmering water and gently slide the egg into the center.

6. Poach the egg for about 3-4 minutes until the whites are set but the yolk is still runny.

7. Use a slotted spoon to remove the poached egg from the water and place it on top of the avocado toast.

8. Season with salt, pepper, and red pepper flakes if desired.

9. Garnish with fresh herbs.

10. Serve immediately.

Prep Time: 10 minutes

Cook Time: 5 minutes

Servings: 1

Lunch: Chickpea and Spinach Salad with Lemon-Tahini Dressing

Ingredients:

- 1 cup canned chickpeas, drained and rinsed

- 2 cups fresh spinach leaves

- 1/4 cup diced cucumber

- 1/4 cup halved cherry tomatoes

- 2 tablespoons sliced Kalamata olives

- 1 tablespoon chopped red onion

- 1 tablespoon chopped fresh parsley

- 2 tablespoons tahini

- 1 tablespoon lemon juice

- 1 clove garlic, minced

- 2 tablespoons water

- Salt and pepper to taste

Preparation:

1. In a large bowl, combine chickpeas, spinach leaves, diced cucumber, halved cherry tomatoes, sliced Kalamata olives, chopped red onion, and chopped fresh parsley.

2. In a small bowl, whisk together tahini, lemon juice, minced garlic, water, salt, and pepper to make the dressing.

3. Drizzle the dressing over the salad and toss gently to coat.

4. Serve immediately.

Prep Time: 10 minutes

Servings: 1

Dinner: Baked Cod with Lemon-Herb Quinoa

Ingredients:

- 2 cod fillets

- 1 tablespoon olive oil

- Zest and juice of 1 lemon

- 1 teaspoon dried thyme

- 1 teaspoon dried parsley

- Salt and pepper to taste

- 1 cup cooked quinoa

- Fresh parsley for garnish

Cooking Directions:

1. Preheat oven to 375°F (190°C).

2. Place cod fillets on a baking sheet lined with parchment paper.

3. In a small bowl, mix olive oil, lemon zest, lemon juice, dried thyme, dried parsley, salt, and pepper.

4. Brush the lemon-herb mixture over the cod fillets.

5. Bake for 15-20 minutes or until the cod is cooked through and flakes easily with a fork.

6. While the cod is baking, prepare the quinoa according to package instructions.

7. Serve baked cod over lemon-herb quinoa.

8. Garnish with fresh parsley before serving.

Prep Time: 10 minutes

Cook Time: 15-20 minutes

Servings: 2

Snack: Carrot Sticks with Hummus

Ingredients:

- Carrot sticks

- Hummus (store-bought or homemade)

Preparation:

1. Dip carrot sticks in hummus.

2. Enjoy as a crunchy and nutritious snack.

Prep Time: 2 minutes

Servings: 1

Day 19

Breakfast: Greek Yogurt Bowl with Mixed Berries and Almonds

Ingredients:

- 1/2 cup plain Greek yogurt

- 1/4 cup mixed berries (such as strawberries, blueberries, raspberries)

- 1 tablespoon sliced almonds

- Drizzle of honey or maple syrup (optional)

Preparation:

1. Spoon Greek yogurt into a bowl.

2. Top with mixed berries and sliced almonds.

3. Drizzle with honey or maple syrup if desired.

4. Enjoy this protein-rich and antioxidant-packed breakfast!

Prep Time: 2 minutes

Servings: 1

Lunch: Quinoa Stuffed Bell Peppers

Ingredients:

- 2 large bell peppers (any color)

- 1/2 cup cooked quinoa

- 1/4 cup black beans, drained and rinsed

- 1/4 cup corn kernels

- 1/4 cup diced tomatoes

- 2 tablespoons chopped fresh cilantro

- 1/2 teaspoon ground cumin

- 1/2 teaspoon chili powder

- Salt and pepper to taste

- 2 tablespoons shredded cheese (cheddar, mozzarella, or your choice)

Preparation:

1. Preheat oven to 375°F (190°C).

2. Cut the tops off the bell peppers and remove the seeds and membranes.

3. In a bowl, mix cooked quinoa, black beans, corn kernels, diced tomatoes, chopped fresh cilantro, ground cumin, chili powder, salt, and pepper.

4. Stuff the bell peppers with the quinoa mixture.

5. Sprinkle shredded cheese on top of each stuffed pepper.

6. Place the stuffed peppers in a baking dish.

7. Bake in the preheated oven for 25-30 minutes or until the peppers are tender and the cheese is melted and bubbly.

8. Serve hot.

Prep Time: 15 minutes

Cook Time: 25-30 minutes

Servings: 2

Dinner: Vegetable Curry with Brown Rice

Ingredients:

- 1 tablespoon coconut oil

- 1 onion, diced

- 2 cloves garlic, minced

- 1 tablespoon grated ginger

- 2 carrots, sliced

- 1 zucchini, diced

- 1 bell pepper, diced

- 1 tablespoon curry powder

- 1 can (14 oz) coconut milk

- 1 cup vegetable broth

- 1 can (15 oz) chickpeas, drained and rinsed

- Salt and pepper to taste

- Cooked brown rice for serving

- Fresh cilantro for garnish

Cooking Directions:

1. Heat coconut oil in a large skillet or pot over medium heat.

2. Add diced onion, minced garlic, and grated ginger to the skillet. Cook until fragrant.

3. Stir in sliced carrots, diced zucchini, and diced bell pepper. Cook for 5-7 minutes until vegetables are slightly softened.

4. Add curry powder to the skillet and cook for another minute.

5. Pour in coconut milk and

vegetable broth. Stir to combine.

6. Add drained and rinsed chickpeas to the skillet. Season with salt and pepper to taste.

7. Simmer the curry for 15-20 minutes until vegetables are tender and the sauce has thickened.

8. Serve vegetable curry over cooked brown rice, garnished with fresh cilantro.

Prep Time: 15 minutes

Cook Time: 25-30 minutes

Servings: 4

Snack: Trail Mix with Nuts and Dried Fruit

Ingredients:

- 1/4 cup mixed nuts (such as almonds, cashews, walnuts)

- 1/4 cup dried fruit (such as raisins, cranberries, apricots)

- 1 tablespoon dark chocolate chips (optional)

Preparation:

1. Mix nuts, dried fruit, and dark chocolate chips (if using) in a bowl.

2. Enjoy as a portable and nutritious snack.

Prep Time: 2 minutes

Servings: 1

Day 20

Breakfast: Banana Walnut Overnight Oats

Ingredients:

- 1/2 cup rolled oats

- 1/2 cup unsweetened almond milk

- 1/2 ripe banana, mashed

- 1 tablespoon chopped walnuts

- 1 teaspoon maple syrup or honey (optional)

- Pinch of cinnamon (optional)

Preparation:

1. In a mason jar or container with a lid, combine rolled oats, almond milk, mashed banana, chopped walnuts, maple syrup or honey (if using), and a pinch of cinnamon (if using).

2. Stir well to combine all ingredients.

3. Cover the jar with a lid and refrigerate overnight, or for at least 4 hours.

4. In the morning, give the oats a good stir and enjoy them cold, or you can warm them up in the microwave if desired.

5. Optional: Top with additional sliced banana, walnuts, or a drizzle of maple syrup before serving.

Prep Time: 5 minutes

Inactive Time: Overnight

Servings: 1

Lunch: Turkey and Avocado Wrap

Ingredients:

- 1 whole grain wrap or tortilla

- 3 oz sliced turkey breast

- 1/4 avocado, sliced

- 1/4 cup shredded lettuce

- 2 slices tomato

- 1 tablespoon hummus (optional)

- Salt and pepper to taste

Preparation:

1. Lay the whole grain wrap or tortilla flat on a clean surface.

2. Spread hummus (if using) evenly over the wrap.

3. Layer sliced turkey breast, avocado slices, shredded

lettuce, and tomato slices on top of the wrap.

4. Season with salt and pepper to taste.

5. Roll up the wrap tightly, folding in the sides as you go.

6. Slice the wrap in half diagonally if desired.

7. Serve immediately, or wrap in foil or parchment paper for a portable lunch.

Prep Time: 5 minutes

Servings: 1

Dinner: Baked Eggplant Parmesan

Ingredients:

- 1 large eggplant, sliced into rounds

- 1 cup whole grain breadcrumbs

- 1/4 cup grated Parmesan cheese

- 1 teaspoon dried oregano

- 1 teaspoon dried basil

- 2 eggs, beaten

- 1 cup marinara sauce

- 1/2 cup shredded mozzarella cheese

- Fresh basil leaves for garnish

Cooking Directions:

1. Preheat oven to 400°F (200°C). Line a baking sheet with parchment paper.

2. In a shallow dish, combine whole grain breadcrumbs, grated Parmesan cheese, dried oregano, and dried basil.

3. Dip eggplant slices into beaten eggs, then coat with breadcrumb mixture, pressing gently to adhere.

4. Place coated eggplant slices on the prepared baking sheet.

5. Bake in the preheated oven for 20-25 minutes, flipping halfway through, until golden brown and crispy.

6. Remove from the oven and top each eggplant slice with marinara sauce and shredded mozzarella cheese.

7. Return to the oven and bake for an additional 10-15 minutes, until the cheese is melted and bubbly.

8. Garnish with fresh basil leaves before serving.

Prep Time: 15 minutes

Cook Time: 35-40 minutes

Servings: 4

Snack: Greek Yogurt with Berries

Ingredients:

- 1/2 cup plain Greek yogurt

- 1/4 cup mixed berries (such as strawberries, blueberries, raspberries)

- Drizzle of honey (optional)

Preparation:

1. Spoon Greek yogurt into a bowl.

2. Top with mixed berries.

3. Drizzle with honey if desired.

4. Enjoy as a protein-packed snack!

Prep Time: 2 minutes

Servings: 1

Day 21

Breakfast: Spinach and Feta Omelette

Ingredients:

- 2 eggs

- 1/2 cup fresh spinach leaves

- 2 tablespoons crumbled feta cheese

- Salt and pepper to taste

- 1 teaspoon olive oil

Preparation:

1. In a bowl, beat the eggs until well combined. Season with salt and pepper.

2. Heat olive oil in a non-stick skillet over medium heat.

3. Add fresh spinach leaves to the skillet and cook until wilted.

4. Pour the beaten eggs over the spinach in the skillet.

5. Sprinkle crumbled feta cheese over one half of the omelette.

6. Cook until the eggs are set and the cheese is melted, then fold the omelette in half.

7. Slide the omelette onto a plate and serve hot.

Prep Time: 5 minutes

Cook Time: 5 minutes

Servings: 1

Lunch: Quinoa and Chickpea Salad

Ingredients:

- 1 cup cooked quinoa

- 1/2 cup canned chickpeas, drained and rinsed

- 1/4 cup diced cucumber

- 1/4 cup halved cherry tomatoes

- 2 tablespoons chopped fresh parsley

- 1 tablespoon lemon juice

- 1 tablespoon extra virgin olive oil

- Salt and pepper to taste

Preparation:

1. In a large bowl, combine cooked quinoa, chickpeas, diced cucumber, halved cherry tomatoes, and chopped fresh parsley.

2. In a small bowl, whisk together lemon juice, olive oil, salt, and pepper to make the dressing.

3. Drizzle the dressing over the salad and toss gently to combine.

4. Serve chilled or at room temperature.

Prep Time: 10 minutes

Servings: 1

Dinner: Grilled Lemon Herb Chicken with Roasted Vegetables

Ingredients:

- 2 boneless, skinless chicken breasts

- 2 tablespoons olive oil

- Zest and juice of 1 lemon

- 1 teaspoon dried thyme

- 1 teaspoon dried rosemary

- Salt and pepper to taste

- 2 cups mixed vegetables (such as bell peppers, zucchini, red onion)

- Fresh parsley for garnish

Cooking Directions:

1. Preheat grill or grill pan over medium-high heat.

2. In a small bowl, mix olive oil, lemon zest, lemon juice, dried thyme, dried rosemary, salt, and pepper.

3. Brush the lemon herb mixture over the chicken breasts.

4. Grill chicken breasts for 6-8 minutes per side, or until cooked through and no longer pink in the center.

5. While the chicken is grilling, toss mixed vegetables with olive oil, salt, and pepper.

6. Grill vegetables for 8-10 minutes, or until tender and slightly charred.

7. Serve grilled lemon herb chicken with roasted vegetables.

8. Garnish with fresh parsley before serving.

Prep Time: 15 minutes

Cook Time: 15-20 minutes

Servings: 2

Snack: Cottage Cheese with Sliced Peaches

Ingredients:

- 1/2 cup low-fat cottage cheese

- 1/2 peach, sliced

Preparation:

1. Spoon cottage cheese into a bowl.

2. Top with sliced peaches.

3. Enjoy as a protein-rich snack.

Prep Time: 2 minutes

Servings: 1

Day 22

Breakfast: Berry Protein Smoothie Bowl

Ingredients:

- 1/2 cup frozen mixed berries (such as strawberries, blueberries, raspberries)

- 1/2 ripe banana

- 1/2 cup plain Greek yogurt

- 1 scoop protein powder (vanilla or berry flavor)

- 1/4 cup almond milk or any milk of your choice

- Toppings: sliced strawberries, blueberries, granola, chia seeds, shredded coconut

Preparation:

1. In a blender, combine frozen mixed berries, banana, Greek yogurt, protein powder, and almond milk.

2. Blend until smooth and creamy, adding more milk if needed to reach desired consistency.

3. Pour the smoothie into a bowl.

4. Top with sliced strawberries, blueberries,

granola, chia seeds, and shredded coconut.

5. Serve immediately with a spoon.

Prep Time: 5 minutes

Servings: 1

Lunch: Chickpea Salad Sandwich

Ingredients:

- 1/2 cup canned chickpeas, drained and rinsed

- 1 tablespoon plain Greek yogurt

- 1 teaspoon Dijon mustard

- 1 tablespoon chopped celery

- 1 tablespoon chopped red onion

- Salt and pepper to taste

- 2 slices whole grain bread

- Lettuce leaves and sliced tomato for serving

Preparation:

1. In a bowl, mash the chickpeas with a fork until slightly chunky.

2. Stir in Greek yogurt, Dijon mustard, chopped celery, chopped red onion, salt, and pepper.

3. Spread the chickpea salad onto one slice of whole grain bread.

4. Top with lettuce leaves, sliced tomato, and the other slice of bread to make a sandwich.

5. Slice the sandwich in half if desired.

6. Serve immediately, or wrap in foil or parchment paper for a portable lunch.

Prep Time: 10 minutes

Servings: 1

Dinner: Salmon with Roasted Asparagus and Quinoa

Ingredients:

- 2 salmon fillets

- 1 tablespoon olive oil

- 1 tablespoon lemon juice

- 1 teaspoon Dijon mustard

- 1 clove garlic, minced

- Salt and pepper to taste

- 1 bunch asparagus, trimmed

- 1 tablespoon balsamic vinegar

- 1 cup cooked quinoa

- Fresh dill for garnish

Cooking Directions:

1. Preheat oven to 400°F (200°C).

2. In a small bowl, whisk together olive oil, lemon juice, Dijon mustard, minced garlic, salt, and pepper.

3. Place salmon fillets on a baking sheet lined with parchment paper.

4. Brush the salmon fillets with the olive oil mixture.

5. Arrange trimmed asparagus on the same baking sheet. Drizzle with balsamic vinegar.

6. Roast in the preheated oven for 12-15 minutes, or until salmon is cooked through and asparagus is tender.

7. Serve salmon and roasted asparagus over cooked quinoa.

8. Garnish with fresh dill before serving.

Prep Time: 10 minutes

Cook Time: 12-15 minutes

Servings: 2

Snack: Apple Slices with Almond Butter

Ingredients:

- 1 apple, sliced

- 2 tablespoons almond butter

Preparation:

1. Spread almond butter on apple slices.

2. Enjoy as a delicious and nutritious snack.

Day 23

Breakfast: Veggie Scramble with Whole Grain Toast

Ingredients:

- 2 eggs

- 1/4 cup diced bell peppers (any color)

- 1/4 cup diced onions

- 1/4 cup diced tomatoes

- Handful of spinach leaves

- Salt and pepper to taste

- 1 teaspoon olive oil

- 2 slices whole grain bread, toasted

Preparation:

1. In a bowl, beat the eggs until well combined. Season with salt and pepper.

Prep Time: 2 minutes

Servings: 1

2. Heat olive oil in a skillet over medium heat.

3. Add diced bell peppers and onions to the skillet. Cook until softened.

4. Stir in diced tomatoes and spinach leaves. Cook until spinach is wilted.

5. Pour the beaten eggs over the cooked vegetables in the skillet.

6. Cook, stirring occasionally, until the eggs are scrambled and cooked through.

7. Serve the veggie scramble with toasted whole grain bread.

Prep Time: 10 minutes

Cook Time: 5 minutes

Servings: 1

Lunch: Turkey and Quinoa Stuffed Bell Peppers

Ingredients:

- 2 large bell peppers (any color)

- 1/2 cup cooked quinoa

- 3 oz cooked turkey breast, diced

- 1/4 cup diced tomatoes

- 2 tablespoons chopped fresh parsley

- Salt and pepper to taste

- 2 tablespoons shredded cheese (cheddar, mozzarella, or your choice)

Preparation:

1. Preheat oven to 375°F (190°C).

2. Cut the tops off the bell peppers and remove the seeds and membranes.

3. In a bowl, mix cooked quinoa, diced turkey breast, diced tomatoes, chopped fresh parsley, salt, and pepper.

4. Stuff the bell peppers with the quinoa and turkey mixture.

5. Sprinkle shredded cheese on top of each stuffed pepper.

6. Place the stuffed peppers in a baking dish.

7. Bake in the preheated oven for 25-30 minutes or until the peppers are tender and the cheese is melted and bubbly.

8. Serve hot.

Prep Time: 15 minutes

Cook Time: 25-30 minutes

Servings: 2

Dinner: Lentil and Vegetable Stir-Fry with Brown Rice

Ingredients:

- 1 cup cooked brown rice

- 1 tablespoon olive oil

- 1 onion, thinly sliced

- 2 cloves garlic, minced

- 1 bell pepper, thinly sliced

- 1 zucchini, thinly sliced

- 1 carrot, thinly sliced

- 1 cup cooked lentils

- 2 tablespoons low-sodium soy sauce

- 1 tablespoon rice vinegar

- 1 teaspoon sesame oil

- Sesame seeds for garnish (optional)

- Sliced green onions for garnish (optional)

Cooking Directions:

1. Heat olive oil in a large skillet or wok over medium-high heat.

2. Add sliced onion and minced garlic to the skillet. Cook until fragrant.

3. Add sliced bell pepper, zucchini, and carrot to the skillet. Stir-fry until vegetables are tender-crisp.

4. Stir in cooked lentils, cooked brown rice, low-sodium soy sauce, rice vinegar, and sesame oil. Cook for another 2-3 minutes, stirring constantly.

5. Remove from heat and garnish with sesame seeds and sliced green onions if desired.

6. Serve hot.

Prep Time: 15 minutes

Cook Time: 15 minutes

Servings: 2

Snack: Greek Yogurt with Honey and Almonds

Ingredients:

- 1/2 cup plain Greek yogurt

- 1 tablespoon honey

- 1 tablespoon sliced almonds

Preparation:

1. Spoon Greek yogurt into a bowl.

2. Drizzle with honey and sprinkle with sliced almonds.

3. Enjoy as a protein-rich snack.

Prep Time: 2 minutes

Servings: 1

Day 24

Breakfast: Spinach and Mushroom Frittata

Ingredients:

- 4 eggs

- 1/4 cup milk (or dairy-free alternative)

- 1 cup fresh spinach leaves

- 1/2 cup sliced mushrooms

- 1/4 cup diced onions

- Salt and pepper to taste

- 1 tablespoon olive oil

- 2 tablespoons grated Parmesan cheese (optional)

Preparation:

1. Preheat the oven to 350°F (175°C).

2. In a bowl, whisk together eggs, milk, salt, and pepper.

3. Heat olive oil in an oven-safe skillet over medium heat.

4. Add diced onions and sliced mushrooms to the skillet. Cook until softened.

5. Add fresh spinach leaves to the skillet and cook until wilted.

6. Pour the egg mixture over the cooked vegetables in the skillet.

7. Cook for a few minutes until the edges start to set.

8. Transfer the skillet to the preheated oven and bake for 10-12 minutes, or until the frittata is set in the center.

9. If desired, sprinkle grated Parmesan cheese over the top of the frittata during the last few minutes of baking.

10. Slice into wedges and serve hot.

Prep Time: 10 minutes

Cook Time: 15 minutes

Servings: 2

Lunch: Mediterranean Chickpea Salad

Ingredients:

- 1 can (15 oz) chickpeas, drained and rinsed

- 1 cup cherry tomatoes, halved

- 1/2 cucumber, diced

- 1/4 cup sliced Kalamata olives

- 1/4 cup diced red onion

- 2 tablespoons chopped fresh parsley

- 2 tablespoons extra virgin olive oil

- 1 tablespoon lemon juice

- 1 teaspoon dried oregano

- Salt and pepper to taste

- Feta cheese for garnish (optional)

Preparation:

1. In a large bowl, combine chickpeas, cherry tomatoes, diced cucumber, sliced Kalamata olives, diced red onion, and chopped fresh parsley.

2. In a small bowl, whisk together extra virgin olive oil, lemon juice, dried oregano, salt, and pepper to make the dressing.

3. Drizzle the dressing over the salad and toss gently to combine.

4. Garnish with crumbled feta cheese if desired.

5. Serve chilled or at room temperature.

Prep Time: 10 minutes

Servings: 2

Dinner: Baked Chicken with Sweet Potato Mash and Steamed Broccoli

Ingredients:

- 2 boneless, skinless chicken breasts

- 1 tablespoon olive oil

- 1 teaspoon paprika

- 1 teaspoon garlic powder

- 1 teaspoon dried thyme

- Salt and pepper to taste

- 2 medium sweet potatoes, peeled and diced

- 1 tablespoon unsalted butter (or dairy-free alternative)

- 2 cups broccoli florets

Cooking Directions:

1. Preheat oven to 400°F (200°C).

2. Place chicken breasts on a baking sheet lined with parchment paper.

3. In a small bowl, mix olive oil, paprika, garlic powder, dried thyme, salt, and pepper.

4. Brush the olive oil mixture over the chicken breasts.

5. Bake in the preheated oven for 20-25 minutes, or until the chicken is cooked through and juices run clear.

6. While the chicken is baking, boil diced sweet potatoes in a pot of water until tender, about 15 minutes.

7. Drain the sweet potatoes and mash with butter until smooth and creamy.

8. Steam broccoli florets until tender, about 5-7 minutes.

9. Serve baked chicken with sweet potato mash and steamed broccoli.

Prep Time: 15 minutes

Cook Time: 25-30 minutes

Servings: 2

Snack: Rice Cakes with Peanut Butter and Banana Slices

Ingredients:

- 2 rice cakes

- 2 tablespoons peanut butter (or almond butter)

- 1/2 banana, sliced

Preparation:

1. Spread peanut butter on rice cakes.

2. Top with banana slices.

3. Enjoy as a crunchy and satisfying snack.

Prep Time: 2 minutes

Servings: 1

Day 25

Breakfast: Berry Chia Seed Pudding

Ingredients:

- 1/4 cup chia seeds

- 1 cup unsweetened almond milk (or any milk of your choice)

- 1/2 teaspoon vanilla extract

- 1 tablespoon honey or maple syrup (optional)

- 1/2 cup mixed berries (such as strawberries, blueberries, raspberries)

- 1 tablespoon sliced almonds (optional)

Preparation:

1. In a bowl or jar, mix chia seeds, almond milk, vanilla extract, and honey or maple syrup (if using).

2. Stir well to combine all ingredients.

3. Cover and refrigerate for at least 2 hours or overnight, until the mixture thickens and becomes pudding-like.

4. Before serving, stir the chia seed pudding to redistribute the seeds.

5. Top with mixed berries and sliced almonds.

6. Enjoy this nutritious and fiber-rich breakfast!

Prep Time: 5 minutes (plus chilling time)

Servings: 1

Lunch: Turkey and Avocado Wrap

Ingredients:

- 1 whole grain wrap or tortilla

- 3 oz sliced turkey breast

- 1/4 avocado, sliced

- 1/4 cup shredded lettuce

- 2 slices tomato

- 1 tablespoon hummus (optional)

- Salt and pepper to taste

Preparation:

1. Lay the whole grain wrap or tortilla flat on a clean surface.

2. Spread hummus (if using) evenly over the wrap.

3. Layer sliced turkey breast, avocado slices, shredded lettuce, and tomato slices on top of the wrap.

4. Season with salt and pepper to taste.

5. Roll up the wrap tightly, folding in the sides as you go.

6. Slice the wrap in half diagonally if desired.

7. Serve immediately, or wrap in foil or parchment paper for a portable lunch.

Prep Time: 5 minutes

Servings: 1

Dinner: Quinoa and Black Bean Stuffed Bell Peppers

Ingredients:

- 2 large bell peppers (any color)

- 1/2 cup cooked quinoa

- 1/2 cup canned black beans, drained and rinsed

- 1/4 cup diced tomatoes

- 2 tablespoons chopped fresh cilantro

- 1 teaspoon ground cumin

- 1/2 teaspoon chili powder

- Salt and pepper to taste

- 2 tablespoons shredded cheese (cheddar, mozzarella, or your choice)

- Sliced avocado for serving (optional)

Preparation:

1. Preheat oven to 375°F (190°C).

2. Cut the tops off the bell peppers and remove the seeds and membranes.

3. In a bowl, mix cooked quinoa, black beans, diced tomatoes, chopped fresh cilantro, ground cumin, chili powder, salt, and pepper.

4. Stuff the bell peppers with the quinoa and black bean mixture.

5. Sprinkle shredded cheese on top of each stuffed pepper.

6. Place the stuffed peppers in a baking dish.

7. Bake in the preheated oven for 25-30 minutes or until the peppers are tender and the cheese is melted and bubbly.

8. Serve hot with sliced avocado if desired.

Prep Time: 15 minutes

Cook Time: 25-30 minutes

Servings: 2

Snack: Greek Yogurt with Mixed Nuts

Ingredients:

- 1/2 cup plain Greek yogurt

- 2 tablespoons mixed nuts (such as almonds, walnuts, cashews)

Preparation:

1. Spoon Greek yogurt into a bowl.

2. Top with mixed nuts.

3. Enjoy as a protein-rich and satisfying snack.

Prep Time: 2 minutes

Servings: 1

Day 26

Breakfast: Banana Almond Butter Toast

Ingredients:

- 2 slices whole grain bread, toasted

- 2 tablespoons almond butter

- 1 banana, sliced

- Drizzle of honey (optional)

- Pinch of cinnamon (optional)

Preparation:

1. Spread almond butter evenly over each slice of toasted whole grain bread.

2. Arrange banana slices on top of the almond butter.

3. Drizzle with honey and sprinkle with cinnamon if desired.

4. Enjoy this delicious and energy-boosting breakfast!

Prep Time: 5 minutes

Servings: 1

Lunch: Quinoa Salad with Lemon Herb Dressing

Ingredients:

- 1 cup cooked quinoa

- 1/2 cup diced cucumber

- 1/2 cup halved cherry tomatoes

- 1/4 cup diced red onion

- 2 tablespoons chopped fresh parsley

- Juice of 1 lemon

- 2 tablespoons extra virgin olive oil

- 1 teaspoon dried oregano

- Salt and pepper to taste

- Crumbled feta cheese for garnish (optional)

Preparation:

1. In a large bowl, combine cooked quinoa, diced cucumber, halved cherry tomatoes, diced red onion, and chopped fresh parsley.

2. In a small bowl, whisk together lemon juice, extra virgin olive oil, dried oregano, salt, and pepper to make the dressing.

3. Drizzle the dressing over the quinoa salad and toss gently to combine.

4. Garnish with crumbled feta cheese if desired.

5. Serve chilled or at room temperature.

Prep Time: 10 minutes

Servings: 2

Dinner: Lemon Garlic Shrimp with Roasted Vegetables

Ingredients:

- 8 oz large shrimp, peeled and deveined

- 2 tablespoons olive oil

- 2 cloves garlic, minced

- Zest and juice of 1 lemon

- Salt and pepper to taste

- 2 cups mixed vegetables (such as bell peppers, zucchini, red onion)

- Fresh parsley for garnish

Cooking Directions:

1. Preheat oven to 400°F (200°C).

2. In a bowl, toss shrimp with olive oil, minced garlic, lemon zest, lemon juice, salt, and pepper.

3. Arrange seasoned shrimp on a baking sheet lined with parchment paper.

4. In the same bowl, toss mixed vegetables with olive oil, salt, and pepper.

5. Spread the vegetables on the same baking sheet around the shrimp.

6. Roast in the preheated oven for 10-12 minutes, or until the shrimp is pink and

cooked through, and the vegetables are tender.

7. Garnish with fresh parsley before serving.

Prep Time: 15 minutes

Cook Time: 10-12 minutes

Servings: 2

Snack: Carrot Sticks with Hummus

Ingredients:

- 2 medium carrots, peeled and cut into sticks

- 2 tablespoons hummus

Preparation:

1. Serve carrot sticks with hummus for dipping.

2. Enjoy this crunchy and nutritious snack!

Prep Time: 5 minutes

Servings: 1

Day 27:

Breakfast: Blueberry Spinach Smoothie

Ingredients:

- 1 cup fresh spinach leaves

- 1/2 cup frozen blueberries

- 1/2 banana

- 1/2 cup plain Greek yogurt

- 1/2 cup unsweetened almond milk (or any milk of your choice)

- 1 tablespoon honey (optional)

- 1 tablespoon chia seeds (optional)

Preparation:

1. In a blender, combine fresh spinach leaves, frozen blueberries, banana, Greek yogurt, almond milk, and honey (if using).

2. Blend until smooth and creamy.

3. If desired, add chia seeds and blend for a few more seconds.

4. Pour the smoothie into a glass and enjoy this antioxidant-rich breakfast!

Prep Time: 5 minutes

Servings: 1

Lunch: Turkey and Avocado Salad

Ingredients:

- 2 cups mixed salad greens (such as spinach, arugula, and romaine lettuce)

- 3 oz sliced turkey breast

- 1/4 avocado, sliced

- 1/4 cup cherry tomatoes, halved

- 1/4 cup sliced cucumber

- 1/4 cup sliced bell peppers (any color)

- 2 tablespoons balsamic vinaigrette dressing

Preparation:

1. In a large bowl, toss mixed salad greens, sliced turkey breast, avocado slices, cherry tomatoes, sliced cucumber, and sliced bell peppers.

2. Drizzle with balsamic vinaigrette dressing and toss gently to coat.

3. Serve immediately as a refreshing and nutritious lunch option.

Prep Time: 10 minutes

Servings: 1

Dinner: Baked Salmon with Quinoa and Steamed Broccoli

Ingredients:

- 2 salmon fillets

- 1 tablespoon olive oil

- 1 tablespoon lemon juice

- 1 teaspoon Dijon mustard

- 1 clove garlic, minced

- Salt and pepper to taste

- 1 cup cooked quinoa

- 2 cups broccoli florets

- Lemon wedges for serving

Cooking Directions:

1. Preheat oven to 400°F (200°C).

2. Place salmon fillets on a baking sheet lined with parchment paper.

3. In a small bowl, whisk together olive oil, lemon juice, Dijon mustard, minced garlic, salt, and pepper.

4. Brush the olive oil mixture over the salmon fillets.

5. Bake in the preheated oven for 12-15 minutes, or until the salmon is cooked through and flakes easily with a fork.

6. While the salmon is baking, steam broccoli florets until tender, about 5-7 minutes.

7. Serve baked salmon with cooked quinoa and steamed broccoli.

8. Garnish with lemon wedges before serving.

Prep Time: 10 minutes

Cook Time: 12-15 minutes

Servings: 2

Snack: Greek Yogurt with Berries and Granola

Ingredients:

- 1/2 cup plain Greek yogurt

- 1/4 cup mixed berries (such as strawberries, blueberries, raspberries)

- 2 tablespoons granola

Preparation:

1. Spoon Greek yogurt into a bowl.

2. Top with mixed berries and granola.

3. Enjoy this protein-packed snack with a satisfying crunch!

Prep Time: 2 minutes

Servings: 1

Day 28

Breakfast: Veggie Breakfast Burrito

Ingredients:

- 1 whole grain tortilla

- 2 eggs, scrambled

- 1/4 cup black beans, drained and rinsed

- 2 tablespoons diced bell peppers (any color)

- 2 tablespoons diced onions

- 2 tablespoons diced tomatoes

- 1 tablespoon chopped fresh cilantro

- Salt and pepper to taste

- Salsa or hot sauce for serving (optional)

Preparation:

1. Heat the whole grain tortilla in a skillet or microwave until warm and pliable.

2. In a separate skillet, scramble the eggs until cooked through.

3. Layer scrambled eggs, black beans, diced bell peppers, diced onions, diced tomatoes, and chopped fresh cilantro on the warmed tortilla.

4. Season with salt and pepper to taste.

5. Roll up the tortilla tightly to form a burrito.

6. Serve with salsa or hot sauce on the side if desired.

7. Enjoy this hearty and nutritious breakfast option!

Prep Time: 10 minutes

Cook Time: 5 minutes

Servings: 1

Lunch: Quinoa and Vegetable Soup

Ingredients:

- 1 tablespoon olive oil

- 1/2 cup diced onion

- 2 cloves garlic, minced

- 1/2 cup diced carrots

- 1/2 cup diced celery

- 1/2 cup diced bell peppers (any color)

- 1/2 cup diced zucchini

- 4 cups low-sodium vegetable broth

- 1 cup cooked quinoa

- 1 teaspoon dried thyme

- Salt and pepper to taste

- Fresh parsley for garnish

Preparation:

1. Heat olive oil in a large pot over medium heat.

2. Add diced onion and minced garlic to the pot. Cook until softened and fragrant.

3. Stir in diced carrots, celery, bell peppers, and zucchini. Cook for a few minutes until vegetables are slightly tender.

4. Pour in low-sodium vegetable broth and bring to a simmer.

5. Add cooked quinoa and dried thyme to the pot. Season with salt and pepper to taste.

6. Simmer for 15-20 minutes, allowing the flavors to meld together.

7. Ladle the soup into bowls and garnish with fresh parsley before serving.

8. Enjoy this comforting and nutritious soup for lunch.

Prep Time: 15 minutes

Cook Time: 20 minutes

Servings: 4

Dinner: Grilled Lemon Herb Chicken with Roasted Vegetables

Ingredients:

- 2 boneless, skinless chicken breasts

- 2 tablespoons olive oil

- Zest and juice of 1 lemon

- 1 teaspoon dried thyme

- 1 teaspoon dried rosemary

- Salt and pepper to taste

- 2 cups mixed vegetables (such as bell peppers, zucchini, red onion)

- Fresh parsley for garnish

Cooking Directions:

1. Preheat grill or grill pan over medium-high heat.

2. In a small bowl, mix olive oil, lemon zest, lemon juice, dried thyme, dried rosemary, salt, and pepper.

3. Brush the lemon herb mixture over the chicken breasts.

4. Grill chicken breasts for 6-8 minutes per side, or until cooked through and no longer pink in the center.

5. While the chicken is grilling, toss mixed vegetables with olive oil, salt, and pepper.

6. Grill vegetables for 8-10 minutes, or until tender and slightly charred.

7. Serve grilled lemon herb chicken with roasted vegetables.

8. Garnish with fresh parsley before serving.

Prep Time: 15 minutes

Cook Time: 15-20 minutes

Servings: 2

Snack: Apple Slices with Almond Butter

Ingredients:

- 1 apple, sliced

- 2 tablespoons almond butter

Preparation:

1. Spread almond butter on apple slices.

2. Enjoy as a delicious and nutritious snack.

Prep Time: 2 minutes

Servings: 1